IS VASECTOMY WORTH THE RISK?

A PHYSICIAN'S CASE AGAINST VASECTOMANIA

H. J. Roberts, M.D.

Senior Active Staff Member, Good Samaritan Hospital and St. Mary's Hopital, West Palm Beach, Florida; Director, Palm Beach Institute for Medical Research, West Palm Beach; Diplomate, American Board of Internal Medicine (recertified); Member or Fellow — American College of Physicians, American College of Chest Physicians, American College of Angiology, The Endocrine Society, American Academy of Neurology, American Diabetes Association, American Heart Association, American Federation for Clinical Research, New York Academy of Sciences, American Association for the Advancement of Science, Sigma Xi (honor scientific research society), Alpha Omega Alpha (honor medical society); listed in *The Best Doctors In The U.S., Who's Who in America, Who's Who In The World, Who's Who In Science and Engineering.*

GW00597249

Sunshine Sentinel Press, Inc.
West Palm Beach, Florida 33407

Includes glossary, bibliographical references, and index.
$16.95

ISBN 0-9633260-2-3

Library of Congress
Number 92-64348
TXu 521 971

Printed in the United States of America

Sunshine Sentinel Press, Inc.
P.O. Box 8697
West Palm Beach, FL 33407
FAX (407) 832-2400

TABLE OF CONTENTS

INTRODUCTION 9

I.   Overview 11

II.   "Vasectogate": The Information Blackout 19

III. The Vasectomy Epidemic 33

IV.   The Vasectomy Crusade 37

V.   The Body's Response to Vasectomy 43

VI.   Some Observed Medical Problems After Vasectomy 53

VII. Medicolegal Implications of Vasectomy 73

VIII. Advice and Perspectives for Men
      Considering Vasectomy ....

APPENDIX:
    FOLLOWUP QUESTIONNAIRE AFTER VASECTOMY.....89

GLOSSARY OF MEDICAL AND TECHNICAL TERMS 93

BIBLIOGRAPHY 101

INDEX 113

OTHER BOOKS BY THE WRITER

Difficult Diagnosis: A Guide to the Interpretation of Obscure Illness. Philadelphia, W. B. Saunders, 1958

The Causes, Ecology and Prevention of Traffic Accidents. Springfield, Charles C Thomas, 1971

Is Vasectomy Safe? Medical, Public Health and Legal Implications. West Palm Beach, Sunshine Academic Press, 1979

Aspartame (NutraSweet®): Is It Safe? Philadelphia, The Charles Press, 1990

Sweet'ner Dearest: Bittersweet Vignettes About Aspartame (NutraSweet®). West Palm Beach, Sunshine Sentinel Press, 1992

DEDICATION

This book is dedicated to Muriel Brenner
for her prolonged encouragement
and support of my research activities.

ACKNOWLEDGEMENTS

I am grateful to Shirley Brightwell and Kathleen Brightwell for their secretarial services.

Beatrice Trum Hunter and Esther Sokol provided valuable editing and suggestions.

The following persons, publishers and companies granted permission to reproduce excerpts and figures.

Dr. Nancy Alexander

Contraception

Couple to Couple League International, Inc.

Dr. R. G. Edwards

Family Planning Perspectives (The Alan Guttmacher Institute)

Mr. John J. Fried

Journal of the American Medical Association

Journal of Experimental Medicine

Journal of Reproduction and Fertility

Krieger Publishing Company

Medical Tribune

Medical World News

New England Journal of Medicine

Patient Care (a division of Medical Economics Co., Inc.)

Dr. Arthur M. Sackler

Saturday Review Press

Science

Southern Medical Journal

Dr. David Wolfers

Nature does not forgive ignorance or wrong advice.
Anonymous

With about 50 million couples worldwide relying on vasectomy for fertility control, any uncertainty about its safety is of serious concern.
The Lancet
(Feature 1991)

Despite the lapse of more than 50 years since vasectomy was first performed for surgical reasons, the long-term effects of this procedure have not yet been completely determined.*
Dr. Nancy J. Alexander (1973)

What happens if we physicians are motivated to say something hopeful that turns out not to be true? Will patients continue to believe us? Why should they? The answers to these questions vary with the circumstances, of course. Certainly, the stakes are high — trust and cherished social credibility.**
Dr. Cornelius O. Granai (1992)

INTRODUCTION

This book deals with a highly controversial subject: the potential long-term risks of wholesale male sterilization by vasectomy. It condenses and summarizes my concerns, stemming from three decades of observation and research, for the general reader.

This effort was pursued without any governmental or institutional grant in order to maintain professional autonomy. Similarly, these studies were not prompted or influenced by any political, social or religious organizations having agendas of birth control and family planning.

My prime purpose is to provide men considering vasectomy, as well as other interested parties, with enough facts so that they will be truly informed about the inherent delayed risks....or at least know what questions to ask. Professional experience, coupled with considerable correspondence (Chapter I) and the continued reluctance of other physicians to express — or even consider — these reservations, has convinced me of this need.

Let me cite just one indicator of the existing search for such information: the anguish of parents and grandparents over the poor health of sons or grandsons in the wake of vasectomy. Their apprehension repeatedly surfaced in an extraordinary way whenever their visits in my consultation office became delayed or interrupted. Seeing my previous book on this subject, IS VASECTOMY SAFE? (Sunshine Academic Press 1979), they intuitively took it from the shelf to examine. An ensuing question became almost predictable: "Where can I buy this book, Doctor?" In turn, I inquired about the reason for such interest. Occasionally, the response was dramatic.

An older couple had been under my care for two decades. In reply to the foregoing query, they indicated that one of their sons began having unexplained and profound medical problems several months after vasectomy. The most immediate concern, however, focused upon their other son who was now contemplating such surgery.

I shall try to present the most significant information fairly, and with a minimum of technical language. A short Glossary is included on pages 93-99 to clarify terms that may be unfamiliar.

All statements are believed to have clinical merit and scientific support...direct or indirect. Only a small fraction of the pertinent references appears in the Bibliography. The reader who seeks more details might wish to consult my previous larger text (Roberts 1979).

Much newer information has been incorporated in the present work. It includes an update of my patient data base, and reports published by others since 1980. Both reinforce concern over the near-universal lack of followup seeking possible long-term consequences of vasectomy by urologists and surgeons in their own patients.

This deficiency is underscored by recent reports of the striking increase of prostate cancer 20 years after vasectomy (Giovannucci 1993).

Among the readers of this book, there will probably be some men who have had a vasectomy. They are invited to complete the Questionnaire in the Appendix (pages 89-92), especially when medical problems occurred subsequent to such surgery. If desired, this questionnaire may be completed anonymously. The form should be mailed to

> H. J. Roberts, M.D.
> 300 27th Street
> West Palm Beach, Florida 33407

Individuals who cooperate in supplying their case histories should recognize the value of such data. Although admittedly "anecdotal," these reports serve to counter the information blackout described in Chapter II. Indeed, they may ultimately further forewarn men who face the vasectomy decision.

Many persons have requested a recorded lecture on this subject. My two-hour talk, IS VASECTOMY SAFE? MEDICAL AND LEGAL ISSUES, is available as a set of two cassettes from the Sunshine Sentinel Press, Inc., P.O. Box 8697, West Palm Beach, FL 33407; FAX (407) 832-2400. (The cost is $19.95, plus $3. for shipping and handling.)

> H. J. Roberts, M.D.

I

OVERVIEW

Where attainable knowledge could have changed the issue, ignorance has the guilt of vice.

Alfred North Whitehead

The new idea, like a bright light in a dark place, always disturbs somebody.

Alvin R. Dyer (1991)

A careful physician...before he attempts to administer a remedy to his patient, must investigate not only the malady of the man he wishes to cure, but also his habits when in health and his physical constitution.

Cicero *(On the Orator)*

Because vasectomy involves surgical intervention in a healthy individual, the possibility that it may produce long-term local or systemic diseases, even in a small portion of the population, has been the subject of consideration. There is an obvious need for a thorough investigation on the safety of this procedure.*

P. E. Bigazzi et al (1976)

---

*© 1976 *Journal of Experimental Medicine.* Reproduced with permission.

THE OPERATION

Vasectomy is usually performed in a doctor's office or an "ambulatory" surgical center. The operation consists of tying or cutting the two tubes (each known as the vas deferens) that carry sperm from the testes (Figure I-1).

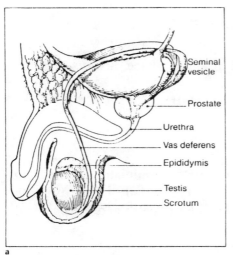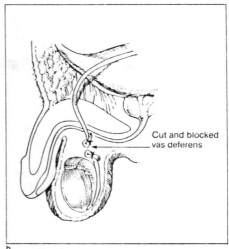

Figure I-1

Anatomy of the male reproductive system (a). The sperm are produced in the testes, stored in the epididymis, and then transferred through the vas deferens to the urethra. Secretions are added en route by the seminal vesicles and the prostate gland. Vasectomy (b) entails the blocking and cutting of each vas deferens.

Vasectomy has received wide acceptance because it is simple, relatively inexpensive, and usually does not incapacitate the person following the operation. Indeed, the "weekend special" consists of having surgery on a Friday afternoon, and returning to work the next Monday.

A number of variations have evolved.

> The "no-scalpel vasectomy" technique has been used extensively in China and Thailand. This method requires two specialized instruments — an extracutaneous vas fixation clamp and a vas dissecting clamp. This rapid and economic alternative to standard vasectomy also eliminates the fear of incisions. Nirapathpongporn, Huber and Krieger (1990) reported that a single physician could perform a daily average of 57 procedures with this method, compared to only 33 procedures using the standard method.

CAUSE FOR CONCERN

Why, then, do I have objections about vasectomy if it is simple, convenient and economical? The answer concerns *long-term safety*. The following statements summarize some basic issues. Each will be discussed in subsequent chapters.

ITEM. <u>Sterilization by vasectomy represents the most widely performed operation ever elected by healthy men</u>... including teenagers (Chapter III).

> *From 10 to 15 percent of all adult men in the United States and Britain have been vasectomized!*

ITEM. <u>Various national organizations, desiring Zero Population Growth (ZPG), champion vasectomy in a crusade-like manner</u> (Chapter IV). Dr. R. K. Daniel (1979) commented: "Currently, the most frequently performed operation in North America is the vasectomy."

ITEM. <u>Profound and permanent changes occur in a majority of vasectomized men</u>. In effect, the man's body becomes allergic — or immune — to his own sperm (Chapter V). In response, several types of antibodies* are produced. Unfortunately, antibodies also have the potential for causing much harm and serious autoimmune disease in some individuals. *I know of no other operation performed on humans that induces responses to such a degree by the immune system.*

ITEM. As a practising physician and medical consultant, I have encountered dozens of relatively young men with otherwise-unexplained diseases — some life-threatening — who had been vasectomized months or years previously (Chapter VI). Since none were aware of my interest in vasectomy as a factor in health problems, they had not sought my consultation for this reason.

ITEM. Similar experiences have been related by physicians, patients and relatives after learning about these possible associations from my writings and previous text (Roberts 1979).

ITEM. Many animal studies have demonstrated changes after vasectomy that are similar to those found in humans.

Unfortunately, most doctors who perform vasectomy remain unfamiliar with this literature. This phenomenon is tantamount to Continuing Medical Ignorance (CMI).

ITEM. Misgivings that I expressed about the potential cancer-causing effects of vasectomy (Roberts 1979, p. 151) have been reinforced by reports of increased cancer incidence in vasectomized men, especially the prostate gland (Giovannucci 1993).

ITEM. Most men requesting a vasectomy are not informed about the preceding information. The vast majority are assured concerning its safety — without any reservations — by their physicians, whom they properly presumed to be experts.

Stated differently, these men were not "truly informed," and their consent was based on incomplete knowledge. Telling the truth to patients, and respecting their autonomy, have become virtual moral absolutes in contemporary American medical ethics. Dr. Edmund D. Pellegrino (1992) asserted

---

*Antibodies are intended to protect against invading foreign substances, whether pollen (as in hay fever), bacteria, or sperm entering the tissues when the sperm-carrying tubes are blocked.

"In this context, truth telling is a necessary corol-
lary, since human capability for autonomous
choices cannot function if truth is withheld, falsi-
fied or otherwise manipulated. Truth telling is
essential to informed consent, the instrument
whereby personal autonomy is expressed in con-
crete decisions."*

ITEM. Every attempt to obtain unbiased "hard data" concerning
the frequency of medical problems among vasectomized
men through serial followup questionnaires (see Appendix)
was rebuffed when I proposed such a joint research venture
with large vasectomy clinics.
Other investigators who were interested in studying related clinical and immunologic aspects in vasectomized
men have encountered similar refusals.

ITEM. A man who wishes reversal of the vasectomy at a later
time, to father more children, is likely to be confronted by
major problems. They include (1) a considerably expen-
sive operation (vasovasostomy), which is generally not covered by insurance, and (2) the high probability that he has
been made permanently sterile (see Chapter VII).

THE URGENT NEED FOR PERSPECTIVE

To repeat: *no other operation performed on humans even
approaches the degree and duration of the multiple immunologic
responses that occur in the post-vasectomy state.* Health professionals and contraceptive advisors must not continue to ignore this
phenomenon, especially for high-risk hyperimmune populations of
developed countries — that is, persons sensitized or rendered allergic to many foreign substances through multiple immunizations
and repeated exposure to environmental chemical and other agents.
In a similar vein, Bigazzi (1981) stressed the need for "caution in
advising this procedure to individuals who may be genetically
predisposed to autoimmune disease."

*©1992 American Medical Association. Reproduced with permission.

In defense of widespread vasectomy, surgeons and public health personnel reflexively refer to published studies that purportedly confirm its safety. After close scrutiny, I have concluded that most protocols of these 'scientific' studies were flawed. For example, one dealt solely with the <u>hospitalization</u> rates for vasectomized men (Walker 1981). The status of out-patient vasectomized men in this group practice, however, was not surveyed — meaning that the majority had been excluded from evaluation.

The ability of <u>one</u> concerned Board-certified internist to find scores of relatively young patients with otherwise-unexplained complications after vasectomy ought not be dismissed casually. It is shortsighted for proponents of vasectomy to denigrate such observations by citing 'a majority of one' because the stakes are too high. Such criticism would be legitimate <u>only</u> if it represents the unadulterated findings of physicians who have <u>carefully</u> and <u>routinely</u> observed the health status of vasectomized men for many years. (I am reminded of the cartoon about a mechanic who stated, "You never know what you'll find once you start looking under the hood.")

PLEAS FOR INFORMATION

I have mentioned my extensive correspondence from afflicted men who underwent vasectomy and members of their family. These letters usually were characterized by attempted objectivity and applied intelligence concerning the problems encountered, extreme frustration with health professionals who had been consulted, and pleas for information.

o A 43-year-old man suffered multiple chronic major illnesses, especially severe joint pain, for 12 years after his vasectomy. He sought help at several pain centers, but in vain. A reversal operation (vasovasostomy) failed to provide relief. He wrote this letter in December 1985.

"The purpose for my letter is to learn if you have obtained any further information that might alter or enhance the findings of your 1979 book. Do you have any new ideas that might lead me out of this painful situation? I would also be interested in the overall reactions you received upon publication of your book. I have personally considered starting a warning campaign to steer others away from this experimental method of birth control. To date, I've been reluctant to take on the main stream medical community."

o The following excerpts are from another correspondent who also developed severe hyperthyroidism (Graves' disease).

"I am writing to you for advice, since your name keeps on popping up as a pioneer in sounding the warnings about vasectomy...I arrived at the conclusion that my "Migratory Arthritis" (my own term) is due to my vasectomy independently of any physician. After arriving at the conclusion that I need a vasovasostomy to reverse my arthritis, I have been laughed at, scoffed at, and ridiculed by a number of physicians, including my urologist, endocrinologist, and regular internist. My hospitalization will not pay for a vasovasostomy unless I can prove it medically necessary. I haven't found a doctor who is willing to so testify ...Can you tell me of any published scientific studies linking arthritis to vasectomy that might help me with my physicians here? Hope springs eternal."

II

"VASECTOGATE"

THE INFORMATION BLACKOUT

I suspect that the outcome of much surgical treatment may be worse than is reported.

A. G. Motulsky (1978)

All professions are conspiracies against the laity.

George Bernard Shaw

Nothing is worse than active ignorance. (Es ist nichts schrecklicher als eine tatige Unwissenheit.)

Goethe

The right to search for truth implies also a duty; one must not conceal any part of what one has recognized to be true.

Albert Einstein

Frustration is experienced by most men who seek in-depth information about the possible long-term hazards of vasectomy in order to make an intelligent 'incision decision.' They are likely to be thwarted in two ways.

First, the individual will be assured—and reassured—by the surgeon or contraceptive counselor that this operation is "completely safe" or "virtually 100% safe."

Second, he will have difficulty in obtaining really pertinent medical and scientific literature. Unfortunately, my attempts to remedy this obstacle, through previous published articles and a book (see Bibliography), had only marginal success.

> The lack of discussion about this issue contrasts sharply with the nearly daily publicity regarding other serious medical or ecological hazards. Numerous accounts concern (1) other types of surgery (e.g., silicone-gel breast implants), (2) reactions to drugs, food additives and pollutants, and (3) a host of threats to health ranging from excessive noise to infant formulas.

This ongoing desire for information about vasectomy continues to be expressed in a stream of thoughtful and provocative letters (Chapter I).

o   One correspondent wrote:
     "I am 34 years old, in excellent health, and seriously considering the procedure. To date I have consulted two urologists, one of whom has undergone the procedure himself. In addition, my wife's gynecologist completely endorses it. However, I am somewhat uneasy that too little followup data have been gathered for most physicians to comment intelligently on the relative safety of the operation. (As an aside, my background includes a B.S. degree in Chemical Engineering and a Masters degree in Business Administration)."

o   A 32-year-old man developed severe allergies for the first time within one month after undergoing vasectomy. He stated:

"Before the operation, I was assured by the literature that a vasectomy is quite painless, and has no risks associated with it. Perhaps my case is rare, but the aftermath of the procedure was very painful for me, and now I am suspicious of the 'low risk' claim."

o   A 32-year-old man wrote:

"I had a vasectomy about 14 months ago. I was concerned at the time about possible negative side effects as I am a bit leery of the medical profession and its invasive procedures, drug therapies, etc. I was assured by my urologist that over 50 years of case studies had shown very little risk or ill effects from vasectomies. I also spoke to several men that I knew who were vasectomized, and other doctors as well about the subject. Nobody I consulted had any major reservations about it. I decided to do it, but in my gut I was concerned about monkeying around with God's handiwork. I have three kids and just didn't even want to take a chance on having another child. I have since been unsure as whether I did something that would cause me trouble (physical or spiritual) later in life...I am very concerned and I need to know the truth. I know other vasectomized men who need to know also. Do you think that the urologists are withholding this controversial information from the public, or are their references just faulty? If I were to contract cancer 10 years from now, for example, how could I prove that the vasectomy was the cause? I hope that I didn't let myself get hoodwinked here as this could be a costly one indeed. Thank you for speaking out. I am eagerly awaiting your reply."

This matter has been reinforced by intelligent professional men who personally related their encounters.

> I was impressed by the convention address of a business writer dealing with creative networking and marketing. We met after this session. On learning of my interest in vasectomy, he volunteered his story.
>
> "I decided to have a vasectomy, and selected a prominent urologist. When I asked about serious complications, he reassured me, in absolute terms, that there was 'no problem.'
>
> "Two days before the scheduled operation, I awoke in a cold sweat. The thought kept recurring: 'This is totally out of character for you because you have not researched the subject adequately!'
>
> "So, at the crack of dawn, I began my <u>own</u> computer search of the medical literature using several major databases. I began with vasectomy in general, and then focused on prostate problems after vasectomy. Guess what? I found <u>three</u> recent articles specifically dealing with <u>cancer</u> following vasectomy!
>
> "I FAXed summaries of these reports to the urologist, and called him. He was not impressed. He then asked, "So, do you want to cancel the surgery?' I replied, 'You bet!'"

THE MAJOR OBSTACLES

Some of the obstacles encountered to obtain factual information about the body's response to vasectomy (Chapter V), and its clinical aftermaths (Chapter VI), will be listed. They constitute other disturbing instances of 'sciencegate' and 'disinformation.'

These encounters by patients recall the assertion by William James: "A great many people think they are thinking when they are only rearranging their prejudices."

'Truth Squads' Attacking 'Anecdotes'

Concerns expressed about wholesale vasectomy, raised by documented reasonable doubts as to its delayed side effects, generally have been ridiculed as "anecdotal" by Zero Population Growth (ZPG) groups and by 'truth squads' of urologists and other physicians. The denigration of observant "anecdotes" in this and other realms is regressive.

o   Dr. Charles Harris (1987) commented:

"But the medical profession has a tendency to discard out of hand, and disparagingly, 'anecdotal' information. Digitalis, morphine, atropine, and the like are chemical derivatives that stem from anecdotal folklore remedies. After all, one anecdote may be a fable, but 1,000 anecdotes can be a biography ...A vital function of the medical profession is to sift the anecdotes and submit them, if possible, to scientific evaluation. But it all starts as anecdote."*

o   The National Research Council (1991) asserted: "Anecdotal reports of neurotoxicity in humans need to be pursued vigorously with clinical surveillance and follow-up."

Absence of Careful and Prolonged Followup

The vast majority of surgeons who contend that this operation is "completely safe" do so without having carefully checked their vasectomized patients over extended periods — that is, at least several years.

Dr. Virginia E. Johnson (1979) appropriately observed: "If you don't want to see it, you won't identify it."

---

*©1987 *Medical Tribune.* Reproduced with permission.

Lack of Familiarity With Existent Literature

Most doctors are not familiar with, or apparently not inter-ested in, the large body of literature regarding changes in both humans and experimental animals after vasectomy (Chapter V). Deficiencies of the articles on which they rely may account in part for such oversight. For example, an extensive review by Mishell (1989) titled, "Contraception," in the *New England Journal of Medicine* did not specifically mention vasectomy or its possible long-term complications.

Superspecialization also contributes to such disinterest, not-withstanding the 'communications explosion.' Many physicians are reluctant to extend their interests into fields other than those directly related to their defined area of involvement. *The Journal of the American Medical Association* (1973; 225:414) editorialized on this phenomenon, which it designated as 'mechanistic isolation-ism.'

> "A man affected with this syndrome gathers infor-mation only on the mechanics of his daily work and forgets a true scientist loves the questions 'Why' and 'By what means?' The specialized reader does not want to dig into Nature's secrets; he does not want to consider his patient as a unit. He becomes, like the orthopedist, a specialist of 'wheel align-ment' who cares little about the engine or other parts of the car. This is an impossible situation to take for a medical scientist. One must be interested in the progress of medicine, in the advance of allied sciences, and dig deep to find what may be of use in daily work."*

Pro-Vasectomy Reviews in *Population Reports*

The November-December 1983 edition of *Population Reports* titled, "Male Sterilization," illustrates institutional blackout of in-formation. (This publication is supported by the United States Agency for International Development.)

o   The 39-page "review," with 560 references, began with this

---

*©1973 *American Medical Association.* Reproduced with permission

summary: "Vasectomy — surgical sterilization for men — is one of the safest, simplest, and most effective methods of contraception. Yet in much of the world, vasectomy is a neglected method...No long-term adverse effects of vasectomy have been observed." (pp. J900-J901)

o   No mention was made of my multiple articles, published letters, and even a book on the negative aspects of vasectomy (see Bibliography).

o   The only pertinent reference appeared under a 'hypothetical effect' of 'immunologic exhaustion.'

"Although preliminary data are reassuring, the long-term effects of vasectomy on immunologically mediated diseases is not known yet. Since these diseases are rare, as many as 10,000 to 20,000 vasectomized men and an equal number of controls should be followed for 10 to 15 years to obtain conclusive results."

Similarly, a discussion of vasectomy in the November-December 1986 edition of *Population Reports*, again focusing on male contraception, stated: "Vasectomy — surgical sterilization for men — is safe, effective, and simple...No long-term adverse effects of vasectomy have been observed."

Failure to Routinely Inquire About Prior Vasectomy

Most physicians do not <u>routinely</u> ask men who present with unexplained medical problems if they had a vasectomy. Some less sophisticated patients even might believe they did not undergo such 'surgery' because they were told that the procedure merely consisted of 'having your tubes tied.' I have encountered this response several times in my practice. An illustration:

A patient experienced a severe syncopal attack. His wife, a registered nurse, noted extreme pallor and a rapid pulse. The attack subsided by the time he reached a hospital. When I saw him in consultation several months later, I detected exquisite tenderness over the deep veins in both calves. At that point, the patient was asked about having had a vasectomy. Replying in the affirmative, he added, "Is that considered an operation?"

Failure of Patients to Admit to Prior Vasectomy

Some men who become ill months or years after a vasectomy may fail to tell their attending doctors about such surgery because they consider it as trivial.

It also is unlikely that most men would connect a present non-urologic problem with prior vasectomy. Therefore, they do not consult the surgeon who performed it.

Failure of Medical Journals to Publish

Few reports that deal with the delayed adverse effects of vasectomy ever appear in widely-read prestigious medical journals. Their editors are reluctant to publish articles, or even brief letters, on this subject for several reasons.

o   The issue may be considered either too controversial or too 'specialized.'

o   The journals may make unreasonable demands for iron-clad statistical validation of clinical observations.

o   Such articles are avoided because they might precipitate law suits, especially relative to the alleged absence of complete informed consent by plaintiffs (Chapter VII).

Flawed Protocols

When asked about possible medical complications after vasectomy, some surgeons cite 'authoritative' reports — e.g., the study by David, de Castro and Mumford (1982) — that appear to absolve the operation. As noted earlier, however, *there were major flaws in the protocols of virtually all such reports*. Every study that I have analyzed regarding the long-range health status of vasectomized men unfortunately had multiple deficiencies in statistical gathering or interpretation.

Giovannucci, et al (1992). A discussion of this statistical long-term study concerning the mortality of vasectomized men is appropriate. It appeared in the *New England Journal of Medicine*. There was a data base of 14,607 men who had undergone vasectomy as of 1976, and 14,607 men who did not have such surgery. The report concluded: "Vasectomy is not associated with an increase in overall mortality or mortality from cardiovascular disease...This study provides reassurance that vasectomy is a safe method of fertility control."

The following comments on this study seem warranted,

o   These men were married to nurses. Accordingly, some confounding variables not mentioned by the authors must be considered. For example, did most of the men — along with their wives — take aspirin daily to prevent a heart attack? (Such medication also might have reduced the incidence of thrombophlebitis and pulmonary embolism.)

o   Did these men adhere to prudent diets (e.g., the minimal use of salt and sugar) and avoid smoking under the continual in-house scrutiny of a concerned health professional?

o   This study focused on heart attack (myocardial infarction) and cancer. No mention, however, was made of thrombophlebitis, pulmonary embolism, serious infections, arthritis, multiple sclerosis, kidney stones, narcolepsy, migraine, allergies and autoimmune disorders, and other conditions encountered after vasectomy (Chapter VI).

o   The data did indicate "an apparent increase in the risk of cancer 20 or more years after vasectomy that requires further study." Specifically, these malignancies included lung cancer, prostate cancer, non-Hodgkin's lymphoma and multiple myeloma. The increase of lung cancer could not be correlated with smoking by the wives, who actually smoked less than the wives of non-vasectomized men in this study (Giovannucci 1992b). These authors later reported a striking increase of prostate cancer (Giovannucci 1993).

Nienhuis, et al (1991). These investigators did a retrospective cohort study using linked medical record abstracts from six health districts in the Oxford (England) region. The data base included 13,246 men aged 25-49 years who had undergone vasectomy between 1970 and 1986, and 22,196 males who had been admitted during this same period for elective operations, appendicitis or injuries. The mean durations of followup were 6.6 years for the vasectomized group, and 7.5 years for the control group.

This report, published in the *British Medical Journal*, concluded that there was no association between vasectomy and an increased risk of testicular cancer or "the other diseases studied." My concerns about the protocol include the following:

o   Hospital admissions and deaths were utilized as the "main outcome measures."

o   Only men who underwent vasectomy on an <u>inpatient</u> or day case basis were selected.

o   There was no detailed interrogation of subsequent illnesses experienced on an outpatient basis.

o   The analysis of subsequent admissions focused on 12 disorders. They did <u>not</u> include multiple sclerosis, thrombophlebitis, pulmonary embolism, infections, psychiatric states, and other problems noted in Chapter VI.

Trivialization of Significant Data

Occasionally, some investigators <u>did</u> find statistically-significant delayed complications following vasectomy — namely, arthritis, connective tissue disease, and prostate or testicular tumors (Chapter VI). In virtually every instance, however, they deemphasized the potential clinical significance of their own findings.

Coercion of Researchers

Some outstanding researchers who studied post-vasectomy phenomena in both man and animals have told me 'off the record' of the extraordinary pressures placed upon them to limit — or even stop — their investigations. Others were coerced to avoid <u>any</u> projections of their major experimental findings onto vasectomized men.

'Negative Reports'

Repeated reference will be made to the 'negative' reports concerning 'alleged' medical complications after vasectomy. For example, the First International Conference on Vasectomy, held at Colombo in October 1982, concluded: "Reassuring evidence that long-term ill effects are not associated with vasectomy" (Davis 1982).

I commented on the 'negative' study by Giovannucci, et al (1992), concerning the apparent absence of increased mortality from cardiovascular disease after vasectomy. This report did not mention a search for other possible complications (other than cancer) listed in Chapter VI. (The bibliography of 44 references failed to include even one of my articles in which they were mentioned.)

Other deficiencies of the "record linkage retrospective cohort study" by Nienhuis, et al (1992) were noted above. It concluded that "we found no evidence to support the hypothesis that vasectomy leads to an increase in the incidence of the various diseases studied."

Disinformation in Patient Education Materials

My review of several all-you-need-to-know 'patient education aids' concerning vasectomy failed to uncover a single specific reference to its potential long-term medical and immunologic complications. One handout asserted that it is "among the safest of surgical procedures." Any mention of potential complications related to the immediate postoperative period — namely, local infection or bleeding, and a localized reaction (granuloma) resulting from the leakage of sperm into the area where the vas was cut.

Inability to Obtain Original Scientific Data

I have repeatedly written the senior investigators of 'case-matched' studies of vasectomized and non-vasectomized men who reached 'negative' conclusions. For example, the report by Massey, et al (1984) titled, "Vasectomy and Health: Results From a Large Cohort Study," involved 10,590 vasectomized men from four cities, with paired neighborhood controls. The conclusion: "Results of this study do not support the suggestions of immunopathological consequences of vasectomy within the period of follow-up." Attempts to obtain the 'raw' data for this study, as well as others, were unsuccessful.

These aspects also are noteworthy.

o   The potential participants were interviewed <u>only once</u> during the <u>five-year</u> study period.

o   Although deaths were recorded, the causes were not published.

o   A number of participants were 'lost.' The authors indicated that "...it may be that as many as one third of the decedent matches were vasectomized."

o   An increased incidence of epididymitis and orchitis (see Glossary) was found.

o   Multiple sclerosis, a disorder having immunological implications (Chapter V and VI), had been diagnosed in <u>nine</u> vasectomized men.

I wrote my congressman: "My concern about the waste of taxpayer monies in funding such studies, when they have not been properly designed or subjected to scrutiny by cooperative scientists whose work is challenged, seems appropriate."

<u>Physician Denial</u>

There is a reflexive tendency of physicians to deny even the possibility of cause-and-effect relationships in certain 'gray' areas. In the case of postvasectomy complications, this unfortunate phenomenon represents the amalgamation of 'brainwashing' and 'complete reassurance by experts.' The following are other examples.

o   There is repeated denial of severe reactions to products containing <u>aspartame</u>, a popular low-calorie sweetener (Roberts 1988, 1989, 1992c).

o   The medical profession's major organizations have failed to express concern about several hazards of <u>fluoridation</u> of public drinking water, especially in the face of widespread intake of considerable fluoride. For example, the vulnerability of fluoridated bone to fracturing has been repeatedly documented (Roberts 1992b).

o   Most physicians and 'nutritionists' adamantly refuse to believe that there are frequent and clinically significant adverse effects due to <u>excessive vitamin E intake</u> (Roberts 1981, 1984).

The following letter from a practising internist illustrates this matter.

> "When I first read your article about vasectomy in the journal *Medical Counterpoint*, I said to myself, 'I had a vasectomy at age 27 and I did not have phlebitis.' But now I recall that about six to twelve months later I noted one morning I could not touch my right heel to the floor without sharp pain in the calf of my leg. Being a physician, I recognized this as a positive Homan's sign (pain experienced in the calf when the foot of a patient with phlebitis [inflammation of the vein] is stretched upward). I then felt the calf of my leg, and it was tender. For about ten to fourteen days I walked around with my heel elevated one or two inches. Finally, I consulted a medical colleague about it. He said I had a mild phlebitis and asked me if I had injured my leg in any way. I searched my memory but could not think of even the slightest injury...
>
> "The reason for the vasectomy was the usual one of wanting to limit my family.
>
> "I thought it interesting that my initial reaction to your article was one of denial of the phlebitis, but it did occur. I felt my case might be typical. I congratulate you on your power to observe."

III

THE VASECTOMY EPIDEMIC

Where there is no vision, the people perish.
Proverbs (29:18)

More is missed by not looking than by not knowing.
Thomas Moore

The Government is very keen on amassing statistics. They collect them, add them, raise them to the nth power, take the cube root and prepare wonderful diagrams. But what you must never forget is that everyone of those figures comes in the first instance from the village watchman, who just puts down what he damn pleases.
Sir Josiah Staamp (1929)

The ultimate significance of any observation can, therefore, be evaluated only over a long period of time. The only advice that can be given is that scientists accept the responsibility of reporting and interpreting their findings in whatever way their best judgement indicates.*
Dr. N. J. Vianna (1975)

GENERAL PROJECTIONS

An estimated 10-15 percent of American men between the ages of 20 and 45 have undergone vasectomy! Stated differently, 15 percent of the partners of all United States women between 18 to 49 years have had a vasectomy (Randall 1992).

Similarly, at least 10 percent of the husbands of women between 25 and 34 years in the United Kingdom consent to vasectomy by the time the wife is 35 (*The Lancet* 1979; 2:1057).

> Confirmation of the fact that about one-tenth of men in the United States and Canada has been vasectomized is found in the Coronary Artery Surgery Study (CASS) data from 14 centers. Of 11,205 men over the age of 30 on whom such information was available, 1106 (9.9 percent) had vasectomies before being enrolled in this study (Kronmal 1988). At different centers, however, the rate ranged up to 25 percent.

Others regard these percentages as underestimations.
o   According to Davis (1982), about 17 percent of married men in the United States between the ages of 35 and 44 had undergone a vasectomy.
o   Federal statistics during 1984 indicated that surgical sterilization surpassed other common methods of contraception. Male sterilization rose from 5 percent in 1965 to 11.2 percent in 1973, and 15.4 percent in 1982 (*The Miami Herald* December 6, 1984, p. A-6).

SUPPORTING DATA

Numerous sets of statistics verify that the numbers of vasectomized men in the United States have escalated over the past three decades. Here are some data:
o   About 12 million men elected vasectomy during the 1970 decade (Alexander 1978).

o   In 1970, a medical marketing and research agency placed the number of annual vasectomies between 699,000 and 750,000. However, these figures did not include vasectomies performed by many private physicians, by public clinics (such as those sponsored by the Planned Parenthood Federation of America), by state institutions, and by the Armed Forces where the extent of vasectomy has been extraordinarily high.

o   In 1970, the number of vasectomies performed exceeded the number of operations for cutting the female tube (tubal ligation).

o   The Association for Voluntary Sterilization estimated that the number of voluntary sterilizations during 1974 was 1,300,000, of which 59 percent were vasectomies — that is, about 682,000 men.

o   During 1980, more than 500,000 men were sterilized by physicians in private practice.

PHYSICIAN 'VASECTOMANIA'

Many urologists and surgeons have met this 'wave of demand' by performing an average of 250 vasectomies a year.

o   One California physician reported to the Association for Voluntary Sterilization that he had done his *ten thousandth vasectomy!*

o   A urologist in Texas informed me that more than 2,600 vasectomies were performed at his clinic — *plus* three or four times that number in his private practice. He was exceedingly proud of the fact that one of his residents could perform 14 vasectomies in less than three hours.

The subject of mass vasectomy in other countries was reviewed in my previous text (Roberts 1979). Reference was made in Chapter I to the nearly doubling of vasectomies performed daily with the 'no-scalpel vasectomy' technique (Nirapathpongporn 1990).

A striking example occurred in Thailand during December 1983 when more than 1,200 men celebrated King Bhumibol Adulyadej's 56th birthday by undergoing free vasectomies. The operation was performed by 50 doctors and 85 nurses at the rate of two men per minute (*The Miami Herald* December 6, 1983, p. A-1). The third most popular song in the country at the time had the title, "I Was Vasectomized."

SOBERING REFLECTIONS

If there is merit to my contention that the 'simple' operation of vasectomy has potentially serious long-term complications, the foregoing figures suggest an incipient major public health problem.

Such concern is magnified by these current phenomena:

o   The superimposed increase of the post-vasectomy load upon other immunologic burdens incurred by numerous environmental chemicals, drugs and immunizations.

o   The enormous social, economic and political repercussions of severely reduced population growth in 'developed' countries.

o   The impressive increase of prostate cancer in vasectomized men, especially after 20 years, as more data have been analyzed (Giovannucci 1993 a, b).

Doubtless, the number of vasectomies will plummet as parenthood continues to decline in middle-class America due to the impact of severe social and economic forces rather than concern about the long-term implications of vasectomy.

IV

THE VASECTOMY CRUSADE

Human history becomes more and more a race between education and catastrophe.

H. G. Wells

Technology now endows an act of irrationality with the greatest of consequences for society.

Dr. Ralph E. Lapp (1973)

Follow-up studies of vasectomy series seem as often as not conducted to show how good the operation is rather than to uncover its effects.*

David and Helen Wolfers (1973)

Valid social ends do not justify invalid, unscientific means...The desirability of zero population growth cannot excuse the routine resort to irreversible, controversial procedures, be they drug or surgical.**

A. M. Sackler et al (1973)

---

*© 1973 *Family Planning Perspectives.* Reproduced with permission of the Alan Guttmacher Institute.
**© 1973 *Science.* Reproduced with permission.

Every man who is considering a vasectomy operation ought to analyze his motivation for this decision. He also should realistically evaluate any added pressures — including patriotism — placed on him (or his wife) by relatives, peers and health professionals. As noted earlier, failure to obtain full and accurate information about the inherent complications of such surgery might result in life-long uncertainty or regret.

Many of the same factors that encouraged millions of men to elect vasectomy in previous generations remain. Some appear even more pressing for today's young couples. They include the considerable expense of having children, limited housing, fears of inflation and recession, the high cost of education, and 'liberation' of women from childrearing responsibilities.

Young couples also are inundated with a barrage of Zero Population Growth (ZPG) propaganda. It ranges from 'people pollution' to 'the ecology.' The frequency of inappropriate and tragically premature decisions to remain childless, or to severely limit the number of children, attest to the effectiveness of such campaigns.

A number of well-known individuals from various fields have lent their prestige to the vasectomy crusade. These notables included Arthur Godfrey, Jim Bouton, Billy Eckstein, Abbie Hoffman, Dean Martin, the Earl of Snowden, Senator Robert Packwood, and Dr. Paul Ehrlich.

Others have commented upon the serious repercussions of these evangelistic efforts. Defending their views on "vasectomania," David and Helen Wolfers (1974) asserted:

> "The quoted passage refers, of course, only to the young, unmarried, childless men trapped into vasectomy by the propaganda efforts of those who (wrongly, in our view) believe they are serving world population or ecological needs by promoting the operation with insufficient discrimination... Unfortunately, the practice of luring young men into vasectomy has been too recently revised for any definite study of its consequences to have been made,

nor should we expect its victims readily to admit their disillusionment."*

The pro-vasectomy literature of *Population Reports*, supported by the United States Agency for International Development, was mentioned in Chapter II. The March 1992 issue titled, "Vasectomy: New Opportunities," reinforced its position in this caption:

"For the man who wants no more children, vasectomy — voluntary male sterilization — offers much: effectiveness, a quick and simple procedure, permanent protection, convenience, little risk of complications, no long-term effect on his own health or sexual performance, and no health risks for his wife."

The publication then asked in bold print: "Why the neglect?" The subsequent section on long-term safety, however, failed to cite even one of my articles or a previous book (Roberts 1979) dealing with potential long-term problems in its bibliography of 208 references.

THE 'CONTAGION OF ACCEPTANCE'

Additional influences have perpetuated the "contagion of acceptance" for vasectomy.

Vasectomy is viewed by many couples as a means of improving their sex life, especially after the age of 35.

Some husbands have a vasectomy to prove they are concerned about the wife's health, presumably based on the contention that "any pregnancy represents a hazard to women."

Men married to wives with a college education are more likely to have a vasectomy when the couple decides upon a course of contraception sterilization.

Widespread concern remains about the side effects of birth control pills (especially when used for long periods), hormonal

---

* © 1974 *Family Planning Perspectives.* Reproduced with permission of the Alan Guttmacher Institute.

injections, and intrauterine devices (IUDs). The number of requests for vasectomy tripled two decades ago following congressional hearings on the possible hazards of some oral contraceptives.

It is recognized that other 'safe' contraceptive techniques are not 100 percent foolproof in avoiding pregnancy.

Coverage for the cost of vasectomy by medical insurance has caused some men to select vasectomy. An arbitrator at Dubuque Packing jested that vasectomies are "at least obligatory as union membership" in light of the fact that more than 300 of its 1,300 unionists chose to have the operation.

Although unofficial, the federal government and several state governments have encouraged vasectomy in several ways.

o   Members of the Armed Forces are readily able to obtain such surgery at most military hospitals and clinics.

o   A law enacted in May 1971 by the Tennessee legislature provided state-subsidized sterilization for anyone unable to afford it.

o   Counseling services for voluntary male sterilization were tax exempted by the Internal Revenue Service (Revenue Ruling 74-595).

The requirements for vasectomy have been liberalized. The Association for Voluntary Sterilization in 1974 conducted a survey of the policies and practices of 56 clinics known to provide vasectomies. The following information was received from 102 clinics (65%) in 38 states:

o   Only about one-tenth of these clinics required the man to be older than 21 years.

o   In 1974, about two out of ten clinics changed the age requirement; more than half lowered it.

o   72% of these clinics would consider a single man of any age as a candidate for voluntary sterilization.

o   64% would sterilize a young husband who was in a childless marriage.

The virtual withdrawal of United States firms from research and development of contraceptive methods (Randall 1992), largely due to tort liability, ensures that emphasis upon vasectomy will

<u>continue for the foreseeable futures</u>. This is clearly demonstrated by their mass exodus from manufacturing intrauterine devices (IUDs) and even contraceptive jellies. In the absence of such acceptable alternatives, many couples are likely to opt for sterilization earlier. This is more true for men because they have few other effective options in controlling their fertility.

V

THE BODY'S RESPONSE TO VASECTOMY

Large long-term follow-up studies are needed to demonstrate the safety of vasectomy in man or to quantify any serious consequences for comparison with the risks and benefits of other methods of contraception.

Editorial, *The Lancet* (1979)

Whatever can happen to one man can happen to every man. (Cuivas potest accidere quod cuiquam potest.)

Seneca

Sit down before fact as a little child, be prepared to give up every preconceived notion, follow humbly wherever and to whatever abysses nature leads, or you shall learn nothing.

Thomas H. Huxley (1825-1895)

Autoantibody formation in many men is due to an obstruction of the vas, leading to the extravasation and resorption of spermatozoa in large numbers. The obstruction can arise in boys or men through vasectomy; greater knowledge of immunology and basic physiological processes, and the availability and purified antigens, should permit constant reevaluation of the dangers and advantages of antibodies.*

R. G. Edwards (1970)

---

* Reproduced with permission.

In discussing the medical conditions I have encountered among vasectomized men (Chapter VI), repeated mention will be made of allergic or autoimmune responses. This review of some pertinent facts and basic concepts helps explain the sequence of events. The Glossary (pages 93-99) further defines medical and technical terms that may be unfamiliar to the general reader.

Concerned persons facing the 'incision decision' also may wish to share and discuss this information with physicians or contraceptive counselors.

THE IMMUNOLOGICAL CASCADE

A. The testes of a vasectomized man continue to make thousands of sperm every minute.

B. These sperm, or their breakdown products, enter the body because the normal barrier between the testes and blood stream is weakened by a buildup of pressure within the severed tubes. The degradation products of sperm, which leak from the reproductive tract in this manner, come in contact with lymphoid tissues. This tends to initiate an autoimmune response.

C. Sperm contain a number of potent antigens—that is, substances to which the body reacts as if they are foreign threats. At least eight human sperm antigens have been identified.

D. Sperm antigens can stimulate multiple antibodies, and alter so-called cellular immunity. These antibodies are known as sperm-agglutinating antibodies, sperm-immobilizing antibodies, and cytotoxic antibodies (see Glossary). A variety of antibodies to the several areas of spermatozoa (acrosome; midpiece; tail) also have been identified. Many of these details were amplified in my earlier text (Roberts 1979).

> The antisperm antibody response has been identified more specifically by newer techniques, such as immunoblotting from two-dimensional gels. Naaby-Hansen (1990) identified five proteins that induced such an antibody (IgM) response in one patient within two weeks after vasectomy.

The antigenic nature of sperm is demonstrated by current efforts to develop a vaccine for women that would prevent sperm from fertilizing an egg (ovum). It takes advantage of the ability of a woman's immune system to develop antibodies to a protein present on the head of sperm at some crucial point in their maturation. Conceptually, such antibodies to sperm will then destroy their ability to fertilize an egg.

E. *A problem unique to vasectomy is the fact that the individual's immune system may not recognize its own sperm.*

F. The production of antibodies following vasectomy commonly persists for prolonged periods, both in man (Figure V-1) and animals (Figure V-2). In one study on rhesus monkeys, an increase in sperm-agglutinating antibody concentrations could be detected seven years after vasectomy. Moreover, these antibodies may persist — or even increase — after the ducts have been surgically reconnected (vasovasostomy).

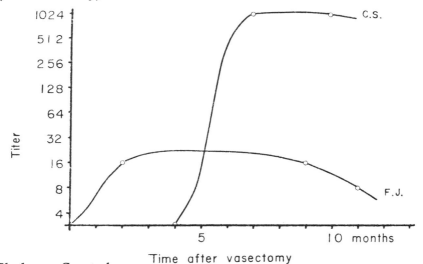

Shulman, S., et al.
Immunologic consequences of vasectomy.
Contraception 1972; 5:269. Reproduced with permission.

Figure V-1

Sperm antibody activity plotted over time after vasectomy in two men. Antibody activity is expressed in terms of sperm-agglutination titer (Kibrick method) in their serum samples.

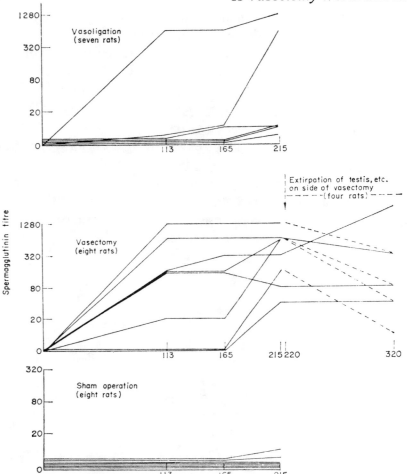

Rümke,P., Titus,M.
Sperm-agglutinin formation in male rats by subcutaneously injected syngeneic epididymal spermatozoa and by vasoligation or
vasectomy.
Journal of Reproduction and Fertility 1970; 21:69-79. Reproduced
with permission.

Figure V-2

Sperm-agglutinin formation after vasoligation (tying the tubes) or
vasectomy (cutting the tubes) in rats.

Shulman, et al (1972) reported sperm-agglutinins in the serum of 55 percent of 22 vasectomized men. Such immunologic activity generally appeared three to six months after surgery; in some cases, it developed as late as the tenth month (Figure V-1). The low titers of sperm-agglutinating activity found in three men prior to vasectomy increased in two after such surgery.

Ansbacher (1977) observed and reported the persistence of sperm antibodies after reopening the severed tubes by a vasovasostomy operation.

"About 50% of men do indeed develop sperm-agglutinating antibodies, and about 25% develop sperm-immobilizing antibodies after vasectomy, with a subsequent fall in antibody titer by 2 years after surgery, but the circulating sperm antibodies do not disappear either with time or after vas reanastomosis [reopening].

"In a series of 15 men followed for at least 18 months after reanastomosis of the vas deferens, circulating sperm-antibody levels rose immediately after the procedure and then fell to the pre-reanastomosis levels by one year after the reversal."

It is of interest that vasectomized men who do not have demonstrable antisperm antibodies in their serum are more likely to show abnormalities reflecting testicular endocrine malfunction (Fisch 1989). These pertain to follicle stimulating hormone (FSH) and luteinizing hormone (LH) activity.

F. *Sperm antigens and antibodies interact. They then may be deposited throughout the body as "immune complexes," and provoke serious reactions within various tissues.* The latter include blood vessels (Figure V-3), kidneys, joints, and even the testes. A host of diseases might ensue.

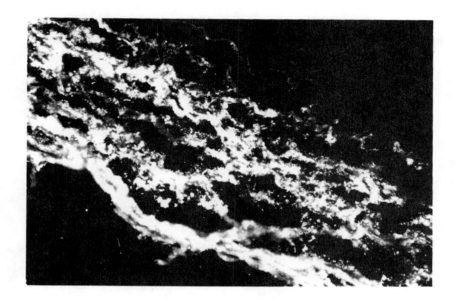

Alexander, N., and Clarkson, T.
Personal communication, April 1978. Reproduced with permission.

Figure V-3

Demonstration of immunoglobulin (IgM) deposition in an atherosclerotic plaque following vasectomy of a *Macaca fascicularis* monkey that had ingested a high-cholesterol diet. This finding was not demonstrable in control animals.

Other investigators have made pertinent observations.

o   Alexander, et al (1986) found a greater incidence and higher levels of circulating antisperm autoantibodies and circulating immune complexes in vasectomized men than in age-matched nonvasectomized controls.

o   Witkin, et al (1982) demonstrated circulating immune complexes from the serum of some vasectomized men, as well as antigens, in about 20 percent of the men tested. (Three different assays were used.) Most of these complexes contained antigen that was reactive with sperm-immunoglobulin; some also contained complement components (see Glossary). These investigators pointed out:

"...the incidence of sperm antibody following vasectomy may have been underdetected. Antibody that was bound to circulating sperm antigen would not react with bound spermatozoa and so would be undetected now in our assay for sperm antibody...Possibly, individuals with a diminished capacity to mount an immune response to spermatozoa may constitute a subpopulation at increased risk following vasectomy."

ADDITIONAL REPORTS ON IMMUNOLOGICAL RESPONSES

Numerous further reports have demonstrated the immunologic aftermaths of vasectomy in both men and experimental animals (Phadke 1964; Rümke 1968, 1970; Ansbacher 1972; Bigazzi 1976, 1977, 1981; Tung 1978). Shulman, et al (1972) commented: "Whether this immune condition spontaneously regresses or instead constitutes an early manifestation of a long-lasting immune process, has yet to be established."

Since the fundamental issue of vasectomy-induced autoimmune responses challenges the safety of this operation, especially for vulnerable subgroups in the population (Chapter VI), several additional studies warrant review.

Mathews, et al (1976)

These investigators reported a significantly higher prevalence of positive autoantibody reactions to multiple antigens other than sperm in 170 men who had undergone vasectomy up to six years earlier, compared with a control group planning to undergo vasectomy. Such autoantibody activity was measured (by indirect immunofluorescence) using various antigens. The latter consisted of liver nuclei, kidney (tubules and brush border), stomach (parietal cells), smooth muscle, and reticulin.

At least one autoantibody reaction occurred in 74.7 percent of vasectomized men, compared with 59.8 percent of men prior to surgery. More positive autoantibody reactions were found among vasectomized men. Also, there was a significant tendency for the proportion of men having at least one autoantibody reaction to increase over time after the operation.

Samuel, et al (1975)

These researchers tested serum from vasectomized men for various antibodies. They reported:

o   55 percent developed agglutinating antibodies.

o   22 percent also developed low titers of antibodies to human protamine. (This is a strong basic nuclear protein that may play a role in the development of autoimmune syndromes by forming antinuclear factors.)

o   22 percent developed cytotoxic antibodies.

o   The presence of antiprotamine antibodies correlated with the presence of agglutinating and cytotoxic antibodies...suggesting that the formation of antibodies against human protamine results from the autoimmune response to spermatozoa.

o   Over time, agglutinins increased significantly in serum. Levels one year after vasectomy were higher than in serum obtained one to four months postoperatively.

Crewe, et al (1976)

Serum from 346 men was analyzed for a variety of nonsperm antibodies before vasectomy and approximately six months thereafter. A positive immunologic response was noted in one or more tests in 96 patients. Autoantibodies were detected in postvasectomy serum — but not in the prevasectomy serum — in 38 patients.

CONTRIBUTORY FACTORS

The immunologic responses to vasectomy by different individuals vary widely — as is true with drugs, food additives, and infectious organisms. This probably accounts for why even more men have not suffered obvious disease after vasectomy.

A number of contributory factors that may increase (or decrease) the response to vasectomy were analyzed in my previous text (Roberts 1979). They include:

o   Heredity
o   Immunizations during infancy and childhood
o   Prior infections, especially by viruses
o   Proneness to allergic reactions
o   Nutritional status (including excessive consumption of calories and sugar)
o   Concomitant hypoglycemia ("low blood sugar attacks") and diabetes
o   Tonsillectomy (involving the removal of important immune cells)
o   Smoking
o   Caffeine abuse
o   The increased "allergic load" resulting from use or exposure to drugs, chemicals, and food additives (e.g., monosodium glutamate; products containing aspartame)

Another variable of possible importance, relative to coronary and cerebral vascular disease (Chapter VI), is the degree of physical activity by vasectomized men. Bridges and Westifield (1984) correlated arterial extensibility with cholesterol deposition in sedentary rats and others that were exercised on a treadmill.

o   The sedentary animals had significantly less extensibility of the aorta.
o   There were significantly increased amounts of cholesterol in the aortic tissue of the sedentary group than in three exercise groups.

VI

SOME OBSERVED MEDICAL PROBLEMS AFTER VASECTOMY

If the clinician, as observer, wishes to see things as they really are, he must make a *tabula rasa* of his mind and proceed without any preconceived notions whatsoever.

J. M. Charcot

At present there is no reason to view vasectomy in the human as a long-term health threat, but I suspect we have not heard the final word on the subject.

Dr. Stephen L. Corson (1983)

Why, even as 40,000 to 50,000 men a year were being vasectomized, did not one bother to carry out a valid set of experiments with either animals or men? Why, for the second time in a little more than ten years, has a contraceptive of essentially uncertain dimensions been unleashed on vast numbers of human beings?*

John Fried (1972)

There are two ways of detecting something that nobody can see: one is to aim at the finest details by getting as close as possible with the best available analyzing instruments; the other is merely to look at things from a new angle when they show hitherto unexpected facets. The former requires money and experience; the latter presupposes neither; indeed it is actually aided by simplicity, the lack of prejudice, and the absence of those established habits of thinking which do tend to come after years of work.**

Dr. Hans Selye (1977)

---

*Fried J. J.: The incision decision. *Esquire* June 1972, p. 120. Reproduced with permission.
** © 1977 Krieger Publishing Company. Reproduced with permission.

My interest concerning the medical complications of vasectomy evolved in an unanticipated manner. Repeatedly, I consulted with relatively young men for a variety of unexplained illnesses, who had histories of such surgery many months or years before the onset of their symptoms. At first, I regarded the association as coincidental. Although I had written several medical texts on diagnosis, I never recalled hearing or reading about these relationships.

As these encounters continued, I began to suspect a legitimate cause-and-effect phenomenon. This inference was reinforced by the fact that most of the men had enjoyed good health prior to vasectomy. As noted previously, none specifically sought consultation because of any awareness of my own interest concerning vasectomy. (These observations were first published a quarter of a century ago [Roberts 1968].)

Subsequently, numerous letters and calls were received from doctors, other health professionals, patients and spouses. All offered impressive accounts of similar or related problems after vasectomy.

To date, this amassed clinical information relates to 74 patients. Twenty-eight of them were seen personally. Information on 46 other persons came from correspondence and details supplied by physicians.

As already noted, the medical and technical language are minimized in this review. Terms likely to confuse nonmedical readers will be defined both here and in the Glossary. More detailed discussions can be found in my prior book, IS VASECTOMY SAFE? MEDICAL PUBLIC HEALTH AND LEGAL IMPLICATIONS (1979). (Available from Sunshine Sentinel Press, P.O. Box 8697, West Palm Beach, FL 33407: $19.95 plus $3.50 for shipping and handling.)

THROMBOPHLEBITIS

Thrombophlebitis refers to the development of a clot (thrombus) in association with irritation of vein walls, usually in the legs and thighs.* This disorder poses two serious problems: (1) local pain, swelling, and severe limitation in walking or standing; and (2) the risk of clots dislodging to the lungs (pulmonary embolism). Thrombophlebitis

---

* Readers may remember thrombophlebitis as a health problem suffered by former President Richard M. Nixon.

often remains "silent" until a pulmonary embolus develops.

Thrombophlebitis occurred in 20 vasectomized men in my series. The post-surgery time ranged from one week to over five years. By <u>routinely</u> asking <u>all</u> patients with <u>thrombophlebitis</u> if they had a prior vasectomy, five men who initially denied such surgery later reported it!

Thrombophlebitis after vasectomy can become a recurring and chronic problem. This was the case with a 27-year-old salesman who experienced recurrent attacks of thrombophlebitis in his lower extremities during the 11 years after a vasectomy, despite many measures, including medications.

Another patient also had repeated attacks of thrombophlebitis involving the upper extremities.

Some of the possible mechanisms for thrombosis in vasectomized men are given below in discussing Angina Pectoris and Myocardial Infarction. An additional factor may be related to the striking increase of thromboxane A_2 by the male hormones testosterone and dihydrotestosterone (Matsuda 1992). This potent constrictor of blood vessels and platelet aggregator appears to play an important role in diseases of the heart and blood vessels.

PULMONARY EMBOLISM

Pulmonary embolism (defined in the preceding section) occurred in 14 patients. This condition is characterized typically by attacks of shortness of breath, pain on breathing (pleurisy), disturbed heart function, and decreased blood oxygenation.

In the patients studied, pulmonary embolism occurred from two weeks to several months or longer after vasectomy. Thrombophlebitis (see above) was present in 10, but undetectable in four by clinical examination and sophisticated testing procedures in my vascular laboratory.

Concern about pulmonary embolism is underscored by one fact: <u>it can be fatal</u>! Indeed, up to 200,000 persons die annually of pulmonary embolism (Roberts 1980). Hence, any condition or operation that initiates or promotes this disorder must be regarded as a potential great threat.

Several patients required heroic measures to the main vein (the inferior vena cava) draining their lower limbs when attacks recurred despite other measures, including the use of blood-thinning medication (anticoagulants). This entailed tying off the inferior vena cava (which requires abdominal surgery), or inserting a sieve-like umbrella through a neck vein.

INFECTION

Serious infections occurred in 20 patients from six weeks to five years after vasectomy, including:

Infection of the prostate gland (recurrent; chronic)	...8
Infection of the epididymis (a tube leading from the testis) — recurrent or chronic	...5
Infection of the kidney	...1
Abscess of the liver	...1
Infection of the blood (bacteremia) and septic shock	...1
Infection of the heart valves (endocarditis)	...1
Recurrent sinusitis	...1
Abcesses of the skin	...1
'Recurrent virus' infection	...1

Multiple and recurrent infections were common in these patients. Other physicians have been impressed by the increased frequency and severity of post-vasectomy infections involving the prostate, epididymis, seminal vesicles (storage glands for sperm near the prostate), and kidneys.

Such susceptibility to infection probably reflects a weakening in the body's immune system caused or aggravated by vasectomy. Also, there may be a cross-reaction between antibodies to bacteria (or other germs) and antibodies to sperm. Professor Gian Franco Bottazzo (1992), Chair of Immunology at the London Hospital Medical College, has championed the view that an "autoimmune virus" heretofore existing symbiotically with humans has become increasingly more virulent.

> This subject provides possible valuable leads concerning the apparent greater vulnerability of homosexuals and prostitutes to human immunodeficiency virus (HIV) infection. One can reasonably hypothesize that repeated exposure to the highly antigenic sperm of many men could alter and reduce their immunologic defense mechanisms. These insights also might be utilized for preparing a more effective vaccine to prevent this ultimately fatal infection.

Although rare, progressively severe and even fatal gangrene has occurred after standard bilateral vasectomy in healthy young men (Viddeleer 1992).

ARTHROPATHY (ARTHRITIS)

A striking feature in nine patients was the recurrence of attacks of severe joint pain and inflammation, and its failure to respond to treatment by many physicians. Multiple joints were involved, especially the wrists, hands, knees and ankles. No patient showed other conventional types of inflammatory arthritis, such as rheumatoid disease and lupus erythematosus.

Two additional patients developed intense back pain due to a severe inflammation of the spine known as ankylosing spondylitis.

Arthritis symptoms were experienced by a 42-year-old man only one week after his vas had been cut accidentally during a hernia repair. Symptoms recurred at least once a month over the next year.

All patients in this category required treatment with a cortisone-like drug, either to relieve acute attacks or as ongoing therapy, due to the frequency and severity of joint pain and swelling.

As with other post-vasectomy complications, this unique arthropathy probably represents an allergic (autoimmune) response to sperm or sperm breakdown products that have entered the body. The ensuing immune complexes (Chapter V) deposited in or near joints can induce inflammation.

Other reports support these observations.

o   One study of the hospitalization rates for a large number of vasectomized men indicated a 2.3-fold increase of admission for arthritis, rheumatism and connective tissue diseases 3 to 5 years after vasectomy, and a 3.7-fold increase nine years or later (Walker 1981).

o   In a questionnaire survey of 4,385 vasectomized men, and 13,155 matched, non-vasectomized controls, Petitti, et al (1982) found a statistically significant association between vasectomy and joint pain or swelling and back trouble.

NARCOLEPSY

Narcolepsy was a prominent feature in 14 vasectomized men. This condition describes an otherwise unexplained state of severe and inappropriate sleepiness. It may or may not be accompanied by other features of the narcolepsy symptom complex. They include sudden attacks of decreased muscle tone during excitement (cataplexy), intensely vivid dreams (hypnagogic hallucinations), and transient muscle paralysis on awaking (sleep paralysis).

In the 14 cases studied, the interval between vasectomy and the onset of pathologic drowsiness ranged from one to four years. Several of these patients sought consultation because of my known interest in this disorder (Roberts 1964, 1967, 1971).

Other doctors have reported intense "fatigue" and decreased activity in patients after vasectomy.

MULTIPLE SCLEROSIS

Five vasectomized men with confirmed or probable multiple sclerosis (MS) have been encountered. This diagnosis was made <u>both</u> by myself and at least one other internist or neurologist. The interval between vasectomy and the initial signs or symptoms ranged from six months to four years.

> The wife of an industrial arts teacher in North Dakota wrote: "My husband had a vasectomy in October 1971. In June 1972, his leg coordination became very poor. After a series of tests, the physicians decided it must be multiple sclerosis."

Goldacre, <u>et al</u> (1979) reported multiple sclerosis in a vasectomy cohort.

It is widely believed that this serious neurologic disease results from changes in the body's immune system. In addition to being provoked by viruses, food, chemicals and other stresses, the antibody responses to vasectomy now must be considered.

MIGRAINE AND RELATED HEADACHES

Attacks of classical migraine and similar "vascular" headaches were the predominant complaints of nine patients. The interval between vasectomy and the onset or aggravation of such severe headaches ranged from one month to several years. Others have reported intensely painful headaches among vasectomized men.

The majority of these patients experienced additional disorders following vasectomy. They included thrombophlebitis, pulmonary embolism, and pathologic drowsiness.

> One correspondent's history included recurrent attacks of headache and thrombophlebitis beginning two years after vasectomy. He was found to have temporal arteritis (inflammation of the superficial arteries in the temple area and elsewhere.)

HYPOGLYCEMIA

Reactive hypoglycemia ('low blood sugar attacks') was a clinical feature in 21 patients. This diagnosis was made on the basis of (1) a history of typical attacks (intense hunger, profuse sweats, tremors, a rapid or irregular pulse, and the inability to think clearly) three to five hours after eating, and (2) their prompt improvement after eating food or sugar. A number of these patients sought consultation with me because of my researches in this area (Roberts 19641,b, 1967, 1968, 1971).

Reactive hypoglycemia was generally confirmed by an appropriate study (the glucose tolerance test). Striking elevation of the blood insulin concentrations often occurred after sugar ingestion. Six patients showed an inability to handle the sugar load properly — a condition referred to as 'chemical diabetes.'

This condition, characterized by the effects of excessive insulin and a severe reduction of energy within the tissues, could contribute to some other problems encountered in vasectomized men. For example, it may aggravate the effects of antibodies and immune complexes (see Chapter V and under "Arthritis"). Further, many changes found in 'chemical diabetes' could adversely alter blood vessels (both small and large), blood clotting, and nerve function. These were detailed in my previous text (Roberts 1979).

ALLERGIC MANIFESTATIONS

The occurrence of disorders suggesting allergic reactions in vasectomized men — most notably, hives (urticaria), swollen tissues in the nose and sinuses, and asthma — is not surprising in view of the persistence of multiple antibodies (Chapter V). The interval between surgery and the onset of symptoms ranged from several months to years.

Eight other men developed rashes that could be considered 'allergic' in nature. (They bear impressive medical names, such as erythema multiforme and erythema nodosum.) Within 10 days after vasectomy, a 30-year-old man developed an extensive rash that persisted for more than a year. He also experienced chronic epididymitis and recurrent 'virus' infections.

The majority of these men and their physicians were perplexed by (1) the explosive onset and persistence of such conditions in the absence of an allergic history, and (2) failure of the symptoms to respond favorably to conventional treatment by experienced allergists. An Ohio correspondent wrote:

"I am 32 years old, trim and healthy, and have always had an extraordinary resistance to colds, viruses, and other diseases. In November of 1978 I had a vasectomy (ligation plus cauterization), and about mid-December developed what I thought was a cold. The condition grew worse. On February 23, I went to a G.P. who informed me that I had an allergy. No medicine seemed to alleviate the symptoms except a very strong turbo-inhalant called Decadron which can be used only briefly because of potentially grave side effects.

"I was sent to an allergist who was very surprised that the allergy occurred so quickly and massively (and in mid-winter) in one who had never had the least problem with allergens. She performed tests, and found that I was allergic to many things in the environment—house dust, mites, dog and cat hair, hormodendrum, grass, ragweed, etc. This news amazed me since I have grown up with pets and other animals, and worked in hay fields and forests with never a trace of congestion; nor do I have a family history of allergies. My condition improved modestly around the middle of this past summer; but I still have a bad case of nasal stuffiness and, because I have a deviated septum, often cannot breathe from one nostril.

"Last spring my wife and I eliminated possible causes of the allergy one by one, and began to suspect the vasectomy as somehow related to my changed condition. Upon researching the field, we found from the latest literature that in most men who have vasectomies, there is an increased production of antibodies, presumably to attack trapped sperm which are theorized to escape into the bloodstream."

An allergist wrote me this letter.

> "I currently have under my professional care a 34-year-old male asthmatic who underwent a vasectomy. His attacks of asthma have progressively increased in intensity and duration over the six months since the operation. He now also has multiple aches and pains, plus occasional attacks of typical erythema nodosum. He does not smoke. He has no known allergies to drugs, foods, or insects. He avoids the use of all alcoholic and carbonated beverages, plus coffee. I feel that my patient is now suffering from some type of an autoimmune reaction after his vasectomy."

Another association with the post-vasectomy state is pertinent when an allergic background was preexistent. Dr. Rudi Ansbacher, a pioneer researcher of sperm antibodies in vasectomized men, used the questionnaire I had devised for studying men after vasectomy. He found a history of allergy in eight of 15 men with sperm antibodies one year following vasectomy, compared to only three of 12 men in whom no sperm antibodies could be detected.

EMOTIONAL DISTURBANCES

Nine patients suffered emotional disturbances — including anxiety, depression, and a sense of sexual inadequacy — following vasectomy. These complaints were sufficiently severe to cause them to seek medical care. The interval since surgery ranged from three months to several years.

Others have reported on the high incidence of post-vasectomy emotional disturbances, even among those previously considered to be well adjusted men.

In one study, Minnesota Multiphase Personality Inventory (MMPI) questionnaires for emotional stability were completed before vasectomy, and again one year after the operation (Edey 1972). The preoperative results had been considered within the normal range. Fifteen of the 35 subjects who completed the second questionnaire evidenced significant personality disturbances.

Admittedly, a convincing case can be made for profound psychological effects inflicted by undergoing a vasectomy. The 'masculine image' may be threatened. (Some women who are sterilized feel less feminine or have lasting regrets about the loss of motherhood.) Additionally, a sense of undue coercion by the wife or a physician to undergo such surgery might be resented.

This 'psychological' conclusion could be wrong, however, in view of the many biological changes that occur in vasectomized men. They include the effects of immune complexes within the nervous system, and altered function of neurotransmitters (chemicals that transmit nerve impulses). I amplified these issues in my previous text (Roberts 1979). Comments by others are pertinent.

o   Dr. Thomas Szasz (1991), a psychiatrist, emphasized: "If mental illnesses are diseases of the central nervous system, they are diseases of the brain, not the mind."

o   Stein, Schiavi and Camerino (1976) stated: "Although clinicians now have an increased understanding of the immunological basis of a variety of illnesses, little attention has been paid to the psychophysiological aspects of immune processes. The immune system plays an important role in biological adaptation contributing to the maintenance of homeostasis [balance] and to the establishment of body integrity."

o   Sydney J. Harris (1983) astutely noted that while technology can protect us from natural perils, it also may be enervating "in the name of restoring us."

IMPAIRED SEXUAL FUNCTION

Markedly reduced sexual drive, including impotence, was a

prominent feature in 11 patients. Three of these men also experienced genital pain on attempted intercourse. One had the left
epididymis removed for postoperative sperm inflammation (granuloma), but the surgery offered no relief.

It is generally held that (1) sexual potency remains unchanged—
or may even increase—after vasectomy, and (2) sexual inadequacy
following such surgery is usually attributable to psychological problems. But it may also be physical. As in the case of emotional
disturbances, discussed above, the explanation might not be so
simple. For example, this operation can damage certain nerves
near the vas that are necessary for proper ejaculation (Alexander
1979). This could account in part for the low fertility rate of men
who have had a vasectomy-reversal operation (vasovasostomy)
(Pabst 1979).

There is a consensus that hormone function generally is unchanged following vasectomy. Yet, by using sophisticated hormonal analysis, significant abnormalities have been found that are
unrelated to the interval since vasectomy.

> Fisch, et al (1989) studied 25 men who had undergone
> vasectomy two to 64 months before investigated. Their
> serum hormone (gonadotropin) responses to gonadotropin-
> releasing hormone were analyzed. The serum follicle stimu-
> lating hormone (FSH) and luteinizing hormone (LH) re-
> sponses were significantly greater in the vasectomy group
> than in age-matched fertile men used as controls. Further-
> more, abnormal responses were more frequent among men
> who did not have identifiable antisperm antibody titers.
> (Serum antisperm antibodies were found in 13 of the
> vasectomized men.)

Infertility After Vasovasostomy

The high incidence of infertility following vasovasostomy is
explained in part by the presence of scarring (interstitial fibrosis)
in the testes noted in vasectomized men by testicular biopsy (Jarow
1985).

Additionally, Linnet, et al (1981) found a strong association between the presence of sperm agglutinins in semen following vasovasostomy, and the impregnation failure of these men for as long as 33 months. Detection of sperm agglutinins in the seminal fluid always was associated with their detection in the serum, usually in a higher titer.

KIDNEY STONES

In an analysis of 1106 men who had a vasectomy before being enrolled in the Coronary Artery Surgery Study (CASS), Kronmal, et al (1988) found a significant increase in the rate of hospital admission for kidney tract stones (urolithiasis). The relative risk was 2.6 for patients 30-35 years old, and 1.3 for those 55-65 years old.

ANGINA PECTORIS AND MYOCARDIAL INFARCTION (HEART ATTACK)

Angina pectoris, myocardial infarction, or both, occurred in four vasectomized men. Two also developed, by months or years, thrombophlebitis or pulmonary infarction — either preceding or following these disorders.

Obviously, one must be cautious before accepting a causal relationship between vasectomy and heart problems in view of the prevalence of coronary disease in our society. A large Seattle study, based upon hospitalization diagnoses, failed to demonstrate any increased incidence of heart attack among vasectomized men. Similarly, Giovannucci, et al (1992a) could not document an increased death rate from myocardial infarction in a large cohort of vasectomized men.

Such epidemiological analyses, however, do not necessarily exclude the role of vasectomy because of (1) flawed protocols, and (2) the inability to focus on individuals due to design of the studies. For example, the incidence of sudden death in non-hospitalized Seattle patients was not published. Similarly, the Giovannucci report did not address several potentially significant prophylactic factors among the husbands of nurses who were studied — e.g., taking aspirin daily, the avoidance of smoking, and adherence to a prudent diet (Chapter II).

The Alexander-Clarkson Studies

This subject, as well as stroke among vasectomized men, will require continued evaluation due to the impressive experimental findings of Dr. Nancy J. Alexander (Oregon Regional Primate Research Center) (1978) and Dr. Thomas Clarkson (the Bowman Gray School of Medicine). They noted that atherosclerosis ('hardening of the arteries') is accelerated in the *Macaca fascicularis* monkey when it ingests a high-cholesterol diet and is then vasectomized. The following observations are noteworthy:

o   Antisperm antibodies developed in all the vasectomized monkeys (as early as 15 days postoperatively), but in none of the control animals.

o   Atherosclerosis was more extensive in the arteries of vasectomized monkeys.

o   An extensive deposition of certain antibodies (known as IgM immunoglobulins) was found in atherosclerotic deposits of the aorta and coronary arteries (Figure V-3).

The recurrent deposition of antigen-antibody complexes tends to injure the lining of blood vessels. This can then set into motion a series of abnormal effects. Alexander and Clarkson suggested that atherosclerosis was initiated and accelerated by sperm antibodies.

Related Observations About Atherosclerosis

Fahrenbach, et al (1980) reported a significant increase of retinal arteriolar constriction in nonhypertensive vasectomized men, compared to matched control subjects. This finding may be relevant to coronary artery disease.

Bansal, et al (1986) studied the long-term effects of vasectomy on experimental atherosclerosis in rhesus monkeys that were observed 18 months on various diets. They concluded that vasectomy *itself* promotes atherosclerosis, especially within the coronary and cerebral arteries.

Jacob (1981) reported another observation relating to accelerated atherosclerosis in vasectomized monkeys. The endothelium (blood vessel lining) of atherosclerotic plaques in these animals contained activated complement components (see Chapter V), as well as sperm antigen. The deposition of such activated complement components could attract and aggregate certain white blood cells (granulocytes), stimulating them to produce toxic oxygen radicals and certain enzymes (proteases). In turn, the latter could damage blood vessel walls, and initiate the development of such plaques.

There is increasing evidence that autoimmune and other mechanisms involved in the development and acceleration of atherosclerosis also may be significant predictors of atherosclerosis, along with smoking and an elevated serum low-density lipoprotein (LDL) concentration. These areas require investigation.

o   An effect on the oxidation of LDL warrants mention because the level of autoantibodies against oxidized LDL has been correlated with progression of atherosclerosis in the carotid arteries (Salonen 1992). An influence of the postvasectomy state on both LDL oxidation and certain endothelial cells lining blood vessels might be conducive to this phenomenon.

o   Vasectomy also may decrease high-density lipoprotein (HDL) cholesterol (Ritchey 1985), which is protective.

o   Vasectomy might influence the several endothelins that exist in large amounts within human seminal fluid (Casey 1992). These 21-amino acid peptides can stimulate the contraction of smooth muscle in many tissues — including blood vessels, the uterus, and the penis (corpus cavernosum).

ADDITIONAL MEDICAL CONDITIONS

Additional disorders occurred in vasectomized patients. Others have made similar observations. For example, vasectomy was linked to kidney stones, arthritis and connective tissue disorders in one study (Walker 1981).

The following list includes otherwise-unexplained medical conditions among vasectomized men in my series.

Number

"Restless legs" 6

Significant weight loss 5

Persistent testicular or scrotal pain 4

Severe leg cramps (at rest)..4

Peptic ulcer, gastritis, pancreatitis 4

Recurrent fever...3

Hypertension 3

Abnormal heart rhythm (arrhythmias)............................3

Generalized glandular (lymph node) enlargement 2

Sarcoidosis (a generalized granuloma reaction)............2

Inflammation or scarring of the lungs 2

Polyneuropathy (irritation of multiple nerves) 2

Inflammation of the kidneys

   (glomerulonephritis; interstitial nephritis)..................2

Aggravation of epilepsy 1

Severe loss of hair (alopecia)..1

Overactivity of the thyroid gland (hyperthyroidism) 1

Air in the chest cavity (pneumothorax) 1

Pancreatitis (inflammation of the pancreas gland) 1

Confusion and memory impairment 1

It is likely that autoimmune responses were involved in many of these cases. Several examples:

o The development of severe hyperthyroidism (Graves' disease) after vasectomy in one patient is relevant because Graves' disease is generally recognized as an autoimmune disorder. The patient also had prolonged testicular pain and "what I call migratory arthritis" involving the left hip, neck, shoulders and low back. (Radioactive iodine treatment was administered.)

o A 43-year-old man had a vasectomy at the age of 29. Subsequently, he developed severe eye problems, a rash on the face, eruption of the mouth, decreased saliva, marked weight loss, intense hip and leg pain, and adverse reactions to foods. He tested positive for antinuclear antibody (a test used to identify patients with lupus erythematosus). A test for sperm antibody (see Chapter V) also was positive. The patient underwent reversal of the vasectomy (vasovasostomy), 13 years after it was performed, but without relief of his distress.

The foregoing list of disorders emphasizes the need for careful and periodic study of ALL vasectomized men. Admittedly, this requires time and entails expense in an era when 'cost-effectiveness' for medical care is demanded. In the absence of such a routine effort, however, the statement that vasectomy is 'completely safe' must continue to be challenged.

TUMORS AND CANCER

Two vasectomized men in this series developed malignant diseases.

o   A man who underwent vasectomy in 1976 was found to have a high lymphocyte count one year later — in conjunction with enlarged lymph nodes and a skin eruption. Subsequently, the diagnosis of chronic lymphocytic leukemia was made, followed by chemotherapy.

o   A widow wrote that her husband was found to have cancer of the kidney seven years after a vasectomy. Since he had been well otherwise, both husband and wife felt that the operation probably played a contributory role.

I concede that the link between vasectomy and cancer is controversial. However, this possible relationship must not be ignored. Several related studies suggest cancer-enhancing mechanisms in vasectomized men.

o   Bendich, et al (1976) provided evidence that sperm can invade the body's 'somatic' cells, as well as egg cells in the ovary. When this occurs, several abnormal responses are set in motion that, biochemically, closely resemble those associated with malignant transformation.

o   Ablin, et al (1980) hypothesized that cancer of the prostate can occur after sensitization by spermatozoa penetrating prostatic tissue. Human seminal fluid also may be a contributing factor in the development of prostate cancer.

o   The reduction in prostatic secretion after vasectomy could result in prolonged exposure of the gland to carcinogenic factors within prostatic fluid (Giovannucci 1993a).

o   The cross-reaction of multiple sperm antigens (Chapter V) with tumor-associated antigens may suppress mechanisms for tumor immunosurveillance (Goldberg 1977).

The very nature of sperm cells relative to forming an embryo cannot be ignored. These observations underscore this issue.

o   Embryonic differentiation antigens are expressed on some malignant cells (Coggin 1974).

o   Tumor growth is increased in some animal models after immunization with embryonic tissues (Chism 1976).

o   Sperm cells are known to express antigens capable of cross-reacting with antigens from malignant cells (Goldberg 1977) and embryonic tissue (Gachelin 1977).

The incidence of various tumors and cancer in vasectomized men, or their sexual partners, is unknown. Repeatedly, I have stressed the need for long-term evaluation of such men by professionally neutral observers who do not perform vasectomies (Roberts 1968, 1971, 1979). This conviction is reinforced by several reports.

o   The Boston Collaborative Drug Surveillance Program (Walker 1981) reported a hospitalization rate ratio of 10.3 for benign prostatic tumors the first two years after vasectomy. The rate ratio declined to 1.9 from the sixth to eighth year.

o   There is mounting concern about the apparent increase of prostate cancer among vasectomized men (Rosenberg 1990, Mettlin 1990, *The Lancet* Editorial 1991).

Rosenberg, et al (1990) found an unexpected association between a history of vasectomy and increased risk for prostate cancer. Multiple comparisons had been carried out using data collected from 1976 to 1988 in a U.S. hospital-based case-control study of many diseases and exposures. The age-adjusted relative risk of prostate cancer was 5.3 when noncancer controls were used, and 3.5 when cancer controls were used. Furthermore, the magnitude of the relative risk estimate appeared unrelated to the interval after vasectomy.

o   Dr. Richard Ablin (1981), a researcher at the Hektoen Institute in Chicago, suggested that prostate cancer could be related to the influence of unejaculated sperm.

o   Harris and Scott (1979) raised a possible relationship between cancer of the female cervix and contact with a vasectomized sexual partner. They noted: "After adjusting for number of partners, we found that the relative risk of cervical cancer in women who had only one partner, who had a vasectomy, was 1.17 times that in women with only one partner, who had not had a vasectomy."

o   Thornhill, Butler and Fitzpatrick (1987), associated with the Irish Testicular Tumor Registry in Dublin, suggested the cancer-causing potential of vasectomy. They found testicular cancer in three men, ranging in age from 35-38 years, within two months after vasectomy. (The tumors had mixed elements of seminoma and malignant teratoma.) Additional reference was made to personal communication with another observer having a comparable encounter. These investigators commented: "...it is not unreasonable to deduce that vasectomy may cause accelerated growth in a concomitant testicular tumor. This could relate to the immune processes that occur after the procedure."

o   Goldacre, et al (1979) reported nine malignant tumors in a vasectomy cohort of 1,764 men followed postoperatively for a mean period of 4.6 years. They included carcinoma of the lung (5 cases), nasopharynx, kidney and testes, and one instance of multiple myeloma (a malignant tumor developing in blood-forming tissues).

o   Cale, et al (1990) conducted a retrospective study at a general hospital in Scotland of all patients who developed testicular tumors during the previous decade. The researchers commented: "Our study suggests an association between vasectomy and subsequent development of testicular tumors...We suggest that vasectomy accelerates the development of a palpable tumor from a carcinoma in situ [in place] or that palpable tumors are overlooked at the time of vasectomy." These investigators recommended followup of vasectomized men for 12-18 months after surgery, with special emphasis upon those having persistent testicular swelling.

o   Giovannucci, et al (1992) reported an apparent increased risk of cancer among a large cohort of men 20 or more years after vasectomy. The malignancies included lung cancer, prostate cancer, non-Hodgkin's lymphoma and multiple myeloma. The investigators commented that this phenomenon "requires further study."

o   Giovannucci, et al reported statistically significant increases of prostate cancer in both a large prospective cohort study (1993a) and a large retrospective cohort study (1993b) of vasectomized men in the United States — viz., 10,055 and 14,607 subjects, respectively. The overall risk increased by 56 percent, but rose up to 89 percent among those who had undergone vasectomy 22 years or longer. Such risk did not appear to be related to diet, level of physical activity, smoking, alcohol intake, educational level, body mass index, geographical area or residence, or detection bias in these carefully conceived studies.

The following experimental studies also are pertinent.

o   There is evidence for the concept of enhanced tumor growth as a result of blocking antibodies or tumor-suppressor cells by antigens that may cross-react with tumor antigens (Goldberg 1977).

o   The incidence and size of spontaneously occurring tumors increases in laboratory mice long after vasectomy (Anderson 1983). Furthermore, this increase correlates with antisperm immunity.

VII

MEDICOLEGAL IMPLICATIONS OF VASECTOMY

In the absence of virtually guaranteed restoration of fertility, presumably on the basis of epidemiological studies covering a minimum of two decades, the prospects for widespread dependence on vasectomy reversals are small, whereas the opportunities for malpractice litigation seem limitless.*

Carl Djerassi (1989)

If anything can go wrong, it will.

Murphy's law

Nature has but one judgement on wrong conduct — if you can call that a judgement which seemingly has no reference to conduct as such: the judgement of death.

Oliver Wendell Holmes

Human beings never welcome the news that something they have long cherished is untrue. They almost always reply to that news by reviling its promulgator.

H. L. Mencken

The magnitude of vasectomies performed on healthy young men (Chapter III) continues. Yet, they receive little or no information about the autoimmune responses and potential medical complications of such 'simple' surgery. If the long-term implications were not so serious, some instances reported to me would be comical.

> An attorney called about a 20-year-old client who sought circumcision, but ended up with a vasectomy. The tubes were reopened three days later at a university hospital.

The physician or contraceptive counselor must pay considerable attention to young husbands with one or several children who find themselves under considerable personal and economic stress, and seek vasectomy to reduce such pressures. Failure to recognize that their decision-making capacity could be impaired at such a critical 'passage' in life might generate serious legal ramifications.

> Applebaum and Grisso (1988) reviewed the legal standards for competent decision-making. They include communicating a choice, understanding the relevant information, appreciating the current situation, and rational manipulation of the information.

Physicians who attempt to defuse a man's apprehension about the long-term safety of vasectomy without making an active attempt to ensure proper and fully informed consent, risk exposing themselves to medicolegal problems. The risk obviously will increase if subsequent epidemiologic studies justify the validity of my published concerns. Specific attention is directed to the occurrence of thrombophlebitis, pulmonary embolism, arthritis, multiple sclerosis, coronary attacks, stroke, recurrent infections, and cancer of various organs (Chapter VI).

The failure to discuss alternative approaches and treatments in detail also invites litigation.

The potential limitations and erroneous inferences of epidemiologic and animal studies have been emphasized repeatedly. Expert witnesses for either side of litigation ought to acknowledge these considerations at the risk of damaging their professional reputation as objective scientists. It is important to appreciate that <u>epidemiology deals with population, NOT with individuals</u>.

> Epidemiology has been defined in the legal literature as "the field of science dealing with the relationships of the various factors which determine the frequencies and distributions of certain conditions and diseases in human populations" (788 *Federal Reporter*, 2nd Series, pp. 744).

I elaborated upon these medicolegal considerations in my previous text, IS VASECTOMY SAFE? MEDICAL, PUBLIC HEALTH AND LEGAL IMPLICATIONS (1979).

THE ISSUE OF INFORMED CONSENT

Sufficient information MUST be given patients in order to provide a basis for truly informed consent, even in the case of "minor" surgical interventions. Although vasectomy is widely regarded as a 'simple' and safe procedure, damages may be awarded for its profound and debilitating delayed complications, local or systemic (Chapter VI).

o   In <u>Schloendorff v. Society of New York Hospital</u> (1914), Judge Benjamin Cordozo expressed the right to autonomy by patients in decision-making in this famous commentary:

"Every human being of adult years and sound mind has a right to determine what shall be done with his own body, and a surgeon who performs an operation without his patient's consent commits an assault for which he is liable in damages."

o   In <u>Swaw v. Klompien</u> (1988), an Illinois appellate court ruled that an award of $510,000 was proper for negligence by a surgeon. The vasectomized patient had become a "couch potato" following severe local complications that included prolonged testicular pain and discomfort.

I have reviewed several "Questions and Answers" pamphlets on the subject of vasectomy that are routinely distributed by urologists and surgeons. Most make no mention of the possible long-term systemic complications (Chapter VI).

The Doctrine of Informed Consent

The Office of the General Counsel of the American Medical Association (Devlin 1983) stated:

> "The legal doctrine of informed consent requires disclosure of information material to a decision concerning proposed treatment before the patient's consent is sought... The physician's obligation is to present medical facts accurately and to make recommendations in accordance with good medical practice."

The doctrine of informed consent has become an essential component of the required standard of duty for health care professionals. In essence, *a physician cannot substitute his or her judgment for that of the patient, or legal representative of the patient, without consent being based on the provision of adequate information about a given treatment, alternative treatments, the collateral risks, and demonstration that the person understands such matters in granting permission to perform.*

Without such total authorization, litigation could be initiated on the grounds of negligence and battery. There have been a number of rulings pertaining to this issue — e.g., Scott v. Bradford (1979), Salvo v. Leland Stanford, Jr., University Board of Trustees (1957), and Canterbury v. Spencer (1972).

There are variations in the rulings by different courts pertaining to the frequency and severity of risks from medical or surgical intervention — ranging from relatively minor ones to death. For example, it has been ruled that risk should be disclosed when (1) there is a one percent risk of death or paralysis, as in Bowers v. Talmage (1963), and (2) there is a one percent risk of hearing loss, as in Wilson v. Scott (1967). Accurate epidemiologic studies assume considerable importance in this context.

Expert medical consultation may be required to address the thorny issue of whether an "informed consent form" signed by a patient constituted sufficiently informed consent. If the matter was a casual routine aimed at saving the doctor's time, and if the procedure failed to cover certain highly relevant risks that the consultant routinely addresses in his or her own practice, the legitimacy of such forms could be properly challenged.

> In <u>Begin v. Richmond</u> (1988), an action of alleged negligence, a man stated that he had not been informed of the possibility of spontaneous reopening of the vas (recanalization) after vasectomy. He and his wife were led to understand that there was no risk of failure if an 8-month semen specimen failed to reveal live sperm. The wife then discontinued use of a birth control pill. She became pregnant two and half years later. The Vermont Supreme Court denied a directed verdict for the urologist, and sent the case back for retrial.

There should be unequivocal documentation when a patient waives his or her right to informed consent. This includes the unwillingness of parents, children or legal guardians to serve as surrogates for the patient.

VIII

ADVICE AND PERSPECTIVES FOR MEN CONSIDERING VASECTOMY

The truth is seldom pure and never simple.
                                        Oscar Wilde

Perhaps the doctor's role in fertility regulation will be seen more and more as assisting someone else's choice, but the new perspective still demands an ethical framework. There will always be an obligation to make sure that the individual understands the nature and consequences of his or her choice, that decisions are not made under pressure from anyone else, and that the alternatives have been made clear.
                                        Editorial, *The Lancet* (1977)

Now physicians are finding that a vast number of sterilized patients are regretting the step and are demanding reversals...what is needed now is to foster a responsible attitude toward sterilization throughout the country. It is only fair—to physicians who want to remain on good terms with their patients, to patients who may be victims of misinformation, and to insurance carriers who foot the bill.*
                                        Dr. Niels Laurensen (1979)

When you rise from your book, probe into what you have learned to discover whether there is in it anything you can translate into reality.
                                        Nahmanides

Most persons who read this book probably do so because they, or someone they care about, is giving consideration to vasectomy. Many probably would ask: "Dr. Roberts, could you condense your knowledge, experience and prolonged thought about contraception and sterilization, including vasectomy, into some general advice — and in nonmedical terms — for individuals or couples facing this decision?"

Here is my initial reply: there are no 'simple' universal answers involving these profound commitments in an open society such as ours. Obviously, numerous differences must be considered. They include age, religious beliefs, education, finances, health status of the husband or wife, stability of the marriage, attitudes concerning abortion, and prior parenthood or nonparenthood. Keeping these factors in mind, the following statements seem fair and valid for men contemplating vasectomy.

o   You cannot assume that you and your wife are capable of having children. Infertility afflicts at least one out of six couples who desire children and try to conceive.

The progressive decline of average sperm counts in young men over the past three decades poses is disconcerting. This deterioration probably can be attributed in part to the effects of prolonged exposure to many chemicals in air, water and food.

o   If you are a young married man, you need to clarify your feelings for or against having children in a realistic way. Whenever the desire for a family remains an honest and mature one, you can deal with the negative views of relatives, friends and doommongers.

The matter of having only one child also requires sober reflection. Single children tend to be confronted with unique problems. Furthermore, the loss of an only child returns and reinforces the pangs of childlessness.

o   You must understand that married couples who 'ultimately' plan to have children, but prolong the delay, are often disappointed. Life is unpredictable. Many good intentions about parenthood have been thwarted by subsequent illness (physical or mental), injury, economic reverses, complications of 'the pill' and intrauterine devices (IUDs), political upheavals, and the loss of fertility with aging.

Concern about the increase of serious risks for the sound health of a fetus whose mother is 35 or older also could influence this decision.

o   If you insist upon contraception, first choose methods that are simple, effective and safe. They include the condom, the diaphragm, the cervical cup, and even the rhythm method. Such advice, however, is conditional upon (1) total familiarity with the particular method by one or both partners, and (2) strict adherence to correct technique.

For example, the condom provides high protection, but is often used incorrectly. This problem has been aggravated by needless restrictions concerning the sale, distribution and advertising of condoms. Many men are not familiar with the large variety of available types and styles.

> Since condoms are no longer restricted to hidden locations in drug stores, enterprising businessmen have opened stores and franchise chains that offer thousands of variations in terms of size, color, taste (lollipop condom), and even products that fluoresce in the dark!

o   Your wife should not take 'the pill' without being (1) informed about the numerous serious side effects caused by these hormones, (2) continually monitored by an interested physician, and (3) advised to avoid attempting conception until the drug has been stopped for at least several months. The oral contraceptives should be avoided, or used with extreme care, by certain 'high-risk' women. They include heavy smokers, and persons who have had high blood pressure, inflammation of the leg veins (thrombophlebitis), heart disease, or diabetes.

o   The risks of intrauterine devices (IUDs) must be carefully explained to both spouses. As with the pill, the woman should be monitored by a doctor at reasonable intervals. Serious infections (some life threatening) and sterility have occurred when such advice was lacking or ignored.

The IUD must be removed if there is any suspicion of pregnancy.

o   If you are a single young man, do not consider vasectomy merely for the purpose of securing sexual freedom without first understanding both the lifelong implications and risks involved. They range from contracting more than a dozen venereal diseases to the serious medical and emotional problems discussed in Chapter VI. The seeming benefits may be far outweighed by these potential risks.

o   As a married man, do not undergo vasectomy unless several conditions are met. Reflect that up to six percent of vasectomees eventually seek reversal of the operation for personal reasons—generally divorce and remarriage.

First, you must be given all the pertinent information about this operation, including its possible delayed immunological effects. Such information, along with all alternatives, should be offered in an unhurried manner by a physician or other counselor, so that your consent is truly 'informed.' The report of the Secretary's Commission on Medical Malpractice, published in January 1973 by the Department of Health, Education, and Welfare, stated:

> "Apart from the legal aspects of the doctrine of informed consent, the patient has a right to know what is happening to his body and to participate in decisions about it. A patient who wants the information should be fully informed of the pros and cons of a proposed treatment or procedure. He is entitled to know both the benefits that may be hoped for and the dangers involved, since only in the light of such knowledge can he fairly decide whether or not he wants the proposed treatment...It is the physician's duty to translate technical terms into language the patient can understand so that complete communication can, in fact, be achieved."

Second, you must be <u>absolutely certain</u> about your desire to have no more children. This requires a searching analysis of yourself and of your marriage. Many divorced men who later remarried have sought reversal of vasectomy (vasovasostomy) despite the high cost of such surgery, and its limited success relative to restoration of fertility.

> Dr. Niels Lauersen (1979), Professor of Gynecology and Obstetrics at Cornell University Medical College, commented: "Now physicians are finding that a vast number of sterilized patients are regretting the step and are demanding reversals."*

The growing number of fathers beyond the age of 40 who have added to existing families, or who have started new ones, attests to the accuracy and wisdom of such perspective. The Fertility Statistics Department of the U.S. Census reported that about one in 20 new fathers were over 40, based on 1989 data. This trend has accelerated due to longer engagements, postponed pregnancies, and the greater patience and focus on the family that comes with maturity.

The significance of antisperm antibodies (Chapter V), in terms of infertility, has been demonstrated from correlations of attempted pregnancy by the partners of men who underwent vasovasostomy. Sullivan and Howe (1977) reported sperm-agglutinating antibodies in 48 percent of such men whose partners became pregnant, and in 94 percent of those who failed to conceive. This suggests the association of an immunological disturbance in cases where the surgery was considered technically successful. It also is consistent with experimental studies linking the failure of female rabbits to conceive after artificial insemination with semen pre-treated with antisperm (whole semen) antibodies (Menge 1971).

Another matter indicates both the probable futility and extreme expense following vasovasostomy even if viable sperm can be demonstrated. Over 100 million dollars are being spent each year

---

*© 1979 *Medical World News*. Reproduced with permission.

at scores of clinics for <u>in vitro</u> fertilization (IVF), which has an estimated chance for success as low as only 14 percent (!) when measured by live births.   Moreover, personal funding is generally required since most insurance companies refuse to pay for IVF. (The latter policy also reflects entrepreneurial abuse in this file.)

     o   <u>If you and your wife believe that there are enough children, and seek contraceptive sterilization without incurring the risks of vasectomy, the best procedure is usually ligation or coagulation of her tubes</u>. Most gynecologists and obstetricians now routinely perform such surgery on an out-patient basis through a small opening in the lower abdominal wall (mini-laparotomy) with minimal complications. It does <u>not</u> risk the medical complications of vasectomy. From a long-term view, the added expense (relative to vasectomy) is not large when one considers the costs of prolonged use of birth control pills and management of their multiple frequent complications.

> There is considerable doubt as to whether the 'tubal ligation syndrome' actually exists. In most instances, pelvic pain, dysfunctional uterine bleeding, abnormalities of menses, or painful intercourse is attributable to other causes (Strickler 1984). They include prolonged use of 'the pill,' and undetected pathology (e.g., uterine fibroids; endometriosis).

The issue of "consent" from one's wife prior to vasectomy tends to elicit disbelief and even off-color jokes in the political context of "equal rights" and a woman's unilateral choice to have an abortion. It assumes more sober overtones if the husband were to suffer chronic medical complications about which the wife had expressed awareness and concern <u>before</u> such "snip, snip, snip" surgery.

     o   <u>Men who decide upon vasectomy ought not place much faith in the 'insurance' of banking their sperm before such surgery</u>. Numerous problems could arise, such as the diminution of stored sperm motility by as much as 90 percent during cryopreservation and entrepreneurial deceit.

SOME LESSONS AND ADVICE FROM
'THE WISDOM OF THE AGES'

Men of all creeds ought to respect the teachings by religious and secular sages in related matters over the centuries. Many concern the old ethical maxim, "Noble goals do not justify ignoble methods." Since the Hippocratic era, the medical profession also has adopted as its motto *primum non nocere — "first, do no harm."*

Responsible young couples should not allow themselves to be misguided by those who preach Zero Population Growth (ZPG) or nonparenthood as a solution to societal ills. This warning assumes particular significance in the face of drastic birth declines within their peer groups.

> Paul Johnson (1987) warned about secular intellectuals who have a passionate attachment to ideas rather than to people in their personal thrust for power. Such collective advice can "often generate irrational, violent and tragic courses of action" when the ideas come before people.

Dr. Herbert L. Fred (1992) related the following appropriate anonymous anecdote in an editorial titled, "Doing Nothing."

> An harassed merchant complained to his rabbi, "I'm in terrible trouble. I can't support my wife and seven children, and every year there comes still another baby. What should I do?"
> After a moment of thought, the wise old rabbi responded: "Don't do anything!"

Dr. Fred commented, "Hurrah for the rabbi!...he took time to think about the matter...For us oldies, doing nothing means doing a lot."

General Guidelines Concerning Contraceptive and Other Technologies

The following commentaries condense many of the author's reservations not only about vasectomy, but also concerning the broad scope of newer technologies. Someone aptly stated: "Wisdom is the ability to discover alternatives."

o   <u>Albert R. Jonsen</u> (1978): "When good persons possess great powers and wield them on behalf of others, they sometimes fail to recognize the harm done as they ply their beneficent craft. The medical profession has such power and its practitioners usually intend to use it well. They must become sensitive to its shadow side."

o   <u>Albert Einstein</u>: "Concern for man himself and his fate must always form the chief interest of all technical endeavors."

o   <u>Charles Frankel</u> (1974): "Technologies of extraordinary power have been turned loose in contemporary society without even the simulacrum of thought about the consequences."

Prayers

A prayer at the beginning of the Jewish Morning Service is remarkably pertinent.

"Blessed art Thou, our God, King of the world, who formed man in wisdom, and created in him various orifices and tubes. Before thy glorious throne, it is revealed that if but one of these be opened or closed, it would be impossible to exist and endure in they presence. Blessed are Thou, O Lord, who heals all flesh and works wondrously."

Vasectomy as a Form of Genocide

Nathaniel Weyl (1967), a scholarly friend, succinctly commented on the disastrous consequences of the failure by gifted married young men with few or no children to reproduce:

"If the father is shot or chooses not to reproduce, the transmission of his abilities or lack thereof is lost to his culture."

Dr. William E. Barclay (1982) editorialized in the *Journal of the American Medical Association:*

"In recent years, a large number of men have submitted to vasectomy to afford themselves greater sexual freedom, but at the cost of permanently imprisoning their genes and consequently making their wives barren."*

SEEKING "THE TRUTH"

A brief commentary on "the truth" seems appropriate. This search remains an ongoing challenge. Zadig, hero of a 1747 Voltaire novelette by the same name, searched for happiness in studying nature — the "great book" — without the bias of prejudice or emotion. This name derives from the Arabic word "saadiq," meaning "the truthful one."

o   Confucius: "Those who know the truth are not equal to those who love it."

o   Thomas Masaryk: "Truth is never in conflict with morality."

o   Maimonides: "No man must surrender his private judgment. The eyes are directed forwards, not backwards."

Embarrassing examples of the elusive nature of "the truth" within nonmedical realms — societal, political, legal, economic, scientific, religious — can be readily recalled. All caution against the legal dictum, "Truth is the ultimate defense." Over the years, such encounters remind me of the quip by some unknown author: "Truth is stranger than fiction, but not so popular."

Flaws continue to be uncovered even in presumably inviolate 'laws of nature,' such as Einstein's theory of relativity. The individuals responsible for them refuse to be diverted from attacking views that they would have preferred to believe...even at risk of being labeled disrespectful or heretical.

I recognize and support the need for family planning and birth control under many circumstances. On the other hand, the election of vasectomy by healthy young men who are not informed of the extraordinary immunological responses to this 'simple' operation, and its potential medical consequences, remains of profound concern to me. The publication of 'scientific' negative rebuttals has not diminished such anguish because careful analysis of their protocols disclosed major loopholes (Chapter II).

---

*© 1982 American Medical Association. Reproduced with permission.

APPENDIX

FOLLOWUP QUESTIONNAIRE AFTER VASECTOMY

This revised questionnaire is used to follow the health status of vasectomized men and control groups.

Readers who have experienced problems after vasectomy are invited to submit the completed form to the address listed in the Introduction.

•　　•　　•　　•　　•　　•　　•　　•　　•　　•

THIS INFORMATION IS CONFIDENTIAL

Present age _____ years

Race (circle)　　White　　Black　　Hispanic　　Asian

Approximate date of your vasectomy operation
Month ____ Year ____

Have you had any of the follotoing medical conditions since your operation?
If yes, please check on the left, and insert approximate dates when they started on the right

	Date
_____ Severe infection (such as pneumonia)	_____
_____ Thrombophlebitis (inflammation or clotting of veins in the legs)	_____
_____ New varicose veins in the legs	

_____Chest pain (please describe below)   _____
_____Palpitations   _____
_____A heart condition (please describe below)   _____
_____Difficulty in urination   _____
_____Inflammation of the prostate gland   _____
_____Unexplained swelling of the feet or legs   _____
_____Pain in or around the joints ("arthritis")   _____
_____Pain on breathing ("pleurisy")   _____
_____Severe tiredness or sleepiness   _____
_____Severe headaches   _____
_____Severe nervousness or tension   _____
_____Marked irritability   _____
_____Severe depression (new; aggravation of
previous depression)   _____
_____Stomach trouble   _____
_____Bowel trouble   _____
_____A growth or tumor (benign or cancer) (please
describe below)   _____
_____A marked gain of weight   _____
_____A marked loss of weight   _____
_____Other operations since your surgery
(please specify below)   _____

Please give more information about the above conditions, and
any other change in your health since the vasectomy operation.
Also indicate whether you were treated by a doctor for them, and if
you had to be hospitalized. (Use the other side of this page, if
necessary)

_____

_____

_____

_____

_____

_____

_____

_____

Did you ever have any of the following conditions *before* your surgery? (circle)

Hay fever	Yes	No
Asthma	Yes	No
Other allergies	Yes	No
Angina pectoris or a heart attack	Yes	No
Migraine headaches	Yes	No
Stomach ulcers	Yes	No
' Diabetes mellitus ("sugar diabetes")	Yes	No
High blood pressure	Yes	No
Hypoglycemia ("low blood sugar attacks")	Yes	No
Phlebitis or thrombophlebitis	Yes	No
Psoriasis	Yes	No
Tonsils removed (tonsillectomy)	Yes	No

Please list *any other* medical conditions you have had

_____

_____

_____

_____

_____

_____

Does anyone in your family have the following conditions? ___
If yes, please circle. Also indicate their relation to you.

			Relationship
Heart trouble	No	Yes	_____
Stomach ulcer	No	Yes	_____
High blood pressure	No	Yes	_____
Arthritis	No	Yes	_____
Diabetes mellitus	No	Yes	_____
Asthma	No	Yes	_____
Other allergies	No	Yes	_____
Psoriasis	No	Yes	_____

Do you take medicine or supplements (vitamins/minerals)?

(circle)   Yes   No

If yes, please indicate which ones.
Medicines _____

_____

Supplements _____

_____

Name (optional) _____

_____

Address (optional) _____

_____

GLOSSARY OF MEDICAL AND TECHNICAL TERMS

abscess—a collection of pus

adjuvant—a substance that leads to a greater immune response when it is mixed with an antigen

agglutinin—an antibody that induces clumping of a particular antigen

aggregation—massing or clumping together

allergy—hypersensitivity to a particular substance

anaphylaxis—a severe allergic reaction to a foreign protein or other substance

anastomosis—the surgical formation of an opening between two hollow tubes or vessels

androgen—a substance that stimulates male characteristics

angina pectoris—acute pain in the chest of a type usually associated with decreased oxygen to the heart

antibody—a protein that is produced in the body in response to invasion by a foreign substance (antigen), and which can react specifically with it

anticoagulant—a substance that inhibits the blood clotting mechanism at some cruical point

antigen—an agent or substance that causes the formation of antibodies

arrhythmia—a variation from the heart's normal beat rhythm

arthropathy—a disorder of the joints

artificial insemination—the instrumental introduction of semen into the female genital tract

aspermatogenesis—the lack of development of mature sperm (spermatozoa)

aspermia—the absence of sperm

asymptomatic—showing no symptoms

autoallergy—autoimmunity or allergic-type responses initiated by processes within the body

autoimmune response—the formation of antibodies directed against the body's own tissues

azoospermia—the absence of sperm in the semen

bacteremia—the presence of bacteria in the blood

bronchitis—inflammation of the bronchial tubes

carcinogen—a substance that can induce cancer

castration—removal of the gonads, resulting in the inability to reproduce

cataplexy—attacks of loss of muscle tone during excitement

cholecystogram—an x-ray study of the gallbladder

chromatin—a stainable portion of the cell nucleus that contains genetic material

colpotomy—an incision in the vaginal wall

complement—a normal component of blood plasma, the presence of which is necessary for many immunological reactions, including antigen-antibody reactions

congenital abnormality—a defect at birth

contraceptive—an agent that diminishes the likelihood of conception

cystitis—inflammation of the urinary bladder

cytotoxic—having a deleterious effect upon cells

dyscrasia—a morbid condition or imbalance

eczema—a skin rash characterized by itching, swelling, blistering, oozing, and scaling of the skin

edema—the abnormal accumulation of fluid

efferent—progressing away from a center or organ

ejaculate—semen expelled in an ejaculation

embolism—the blocking of a blood vessel by a clot or other substance brought there by the circulating blood

endocarditis—an infection or inflammation of the inner lining of the heart or heart valves

endocrine disorders—abnormal functioning of glands that produce hormones

enzymes—substances that initiate and accelerate chemical reactions

epidemiology—the study of factors that influence the frequency and distribution of disease among populations

epididymis—a convoluted tube, as much as 20 feet in length, where matured sperm coming from the testes are stored

epididymitis—inflammation of the epididymis

epilepsy—a convulsive disorder consisting of seizures and diminished consciousness

erythema—congestive redness of the skin

estrogen—a general name for the principal female sex hormones

exogenous—an influence originating outside the body or organism

extravasation—the escape of fluid or other material into the tissues

exudation—the accumulation of fluid which has oozed through the tissues

fertility—the capacity to conceive (induce conception)

fetus—an unborn offspring (in humans, from about eight weeks after fertilization to birth)

fibrosis—the formation of fibrous or scar tissue

follicle stimulating hormone (FSH)—a hormone secreted in the anterior pituitary gland that stimulates the growth and maturation of egg follicles in the ovary, and sperm-producing cells in the testes

glomerulonephritis—kidney inflammation involving the glomeruli

gonad—sex gland

granuloma—a type of inflammatory response in tissues

hepatic—pertaining to the liver

histology—the microscopic study of the form and structure of tissues making up living organisms

homeostasis—a tendency to stability or uniformity in the normal body state

hyperinsulinism—the excessive secretion of insulin by the pancreas, often resulting in hypoglycemia ("low blood sugar")

hyperplasia—abnormal cell growth with an increase in size

hypertension—an abnormal elevation of the blood pressure

hypoglycemia—decreased blood glucose ("low blood sugar")

iatrogenic—a physician-related influence

immune—a response of the organism to elements recognized as foreign (that is, not part of itself)

immunoglobulin—a serum globulin (protein) having antibody activity

immunology—the science concerned with resistance or immunity to disease immunopathology—the study of diseases resulting from antigen-antibody reactions produced by immunologic responses

immunosuppressant—a substance capable of suppressing immune response(s)

impotence—partial or complete inability of the male to perform the sexual act

in vitro—observable in a test tube or other artificial environment

infarction—development of a localized area of dead (infarcted) tissue

interstitial—within the intervals or gaps of a tissue or structure

ischemia—deficient supply of blood to an organ due to obstruction of its blood supply, whether physical closure or severe spasm

laparotomy—opening the abdominal wall

lupus erythematosus—a form of immunologic inflammatory disease causing deterioration of connective tissues, with or without a characteristic rash

luteinizing hormone (LH)—a hormone secreted by the anterior pituitary gland that stimulates the production of corpora lutea in the ovaries after ovulation, and the secretion of testosterone by the testes

macrophage—a large cell or phagocyte that can destroy harmful organisms or foreign material

mean (geometric)—an average between two extremes

metabolic disorder—a disease or health problem resulting from the malfunctioning of the process of transforming nutrients from food for use by the body

migraine—a symptom complex consisting of periodic attacks of severe vascular headaches, often accompanied by irritability, visual impairmant, nausea and vomiting

morbidity—the condition of being diseased; the rate of total number of diseased individuals to the total number of persons in a population

mortality—the ratio of total number of deaths to the total number of persons in a population

motile—having spontaneous movement

multiple sclerosis—a disease characterized by hardened patches (plaques) scattered throughout the brain and spinal cord, which interfere with functions of the affected nerves

mutagenic—inducing a genetic mutation or change

myocardial infarction—the development of dead heart muscle due to interruption of its blood supply

narcolepsy—pathological drowsiness and sleep

necrosis—the death of cells or tissue resulting from disease or injury

oligospermia—a deficient number of sperm in the semen

oncogenic—inducing tumor growth

orchitis—an inflammation of the testis

paresthesia—abnormal sensation due to a disorder of sensory nerves

pathogenicity—the capacity to induce disease

pathologic—pertaining to or caused by disease

phlebothrombosis—the presence of a clot in a vein

pleurisy—an inflammation of the membrane (pleura) around the lung

pneumonitis—an inflammation of lung tissue (pneumonia)

pneumothorax—an abnormal presence of air in the pleural cavity of the chest

polyneuropathy—a disease involving several nerves

prednisone and prednisolone—cortisone-like drugs

prostate—a walnut-sized organ in the male that secretes part of the seminal fluid

prostatitis—an inflammation of the prostate gland

proximal—closest to the point of reference

psoriasis—a chronic recurrent skin disease characterized by bright red patches covered with scales

puerperium—the state after birth

recanalization—reopening

refractory—not readily yielding to treatment

sarcoidosis—a chronic disease of unknown cause that is characterized by inflammatory reactions (granulomas) in many organs

scrotum—the skin covering the testis and epididymis

semen—fluid discharged at ejaculation in the male, consisting of sperm and secretions from the prostate and other accessory sexual glands

seminal vesicles—paired structures in the male close to the urinary bladder that open into the vas deferens

seminiferous tubules—tubules of the testis in which sperm develop, and through which they leave the gland

sepsis—a morbid condition caused by pathogenic bacteria or other infectious organisms in the blood or tissues

somatic—pertaining to, or characteristic, of the body

sperm—the mature germ cell of a male made by the testes

spermatogenesis—sperm production

spermatozoa—mature male gene cells made by the testes that consist of a head (or nucleus), a neck, a middle area, and a tail

sterility—the inability to produce offspring

sterilization—the process of rendering an individual incapable of reproduction

tachycardia—rapid heart action

teratogenic—the ability to produce abnormalities (anomalies) of formation in the developing fetus

testes—organs wherein sperm are manufactured and then mature

testosterone—one of the male sex hormones produced by the testes

thromboembolism—the obstruction of a blood vessel by a clot (thrombus) that has broken loose

thrombophlebitis—the development of a thrombus (clot) in association with inflammatory changes of the blood vessel wall

titer—the quantity of a substance required to react with, or correspond to, a given amount of another substance

tubal ligation—tying of the fallopian tubes in a female to prevent pregnancy

tumorigenic—contributing to the production of tumors

urology—the medical science dealing with the urinary system in the female, and the genitourinary system in the male

urticaria—hives

vas deferens—the straight tube conducting sperm to the prostate gland and ultimately the ejaculate

vasculature—the supply of vessels to a specific region

vasectomy—the surgical interruption of the vas deferens on both
  sides

vasoligation—the surgical ligation of the vas deferens

vasovasostomy—the surgical realignment and reopening of the vas
  deferens

BIBLIOGRAPHY

Ablin, R. J., Bhatti, R. A., Bush, I. M., Guinan, P. D.: Effect of human seminal plasma on tumour-associated immunity in patients with adenocarcinoma of the prostate. *Journal of Reproductive Immunology* 1980; 1:337-345.

Ablin, R.: Cited in *The Evening Times* (West Palm Beach), February 23, 1981, A-12.

Alexander, N. J.: Vasectomy: Long-term effects. *Science* 1973; 182:946.

Alexander, N., Clarkson, T. B.: Cited by *Medical Tribune*, June 7, 1978, 1.

Alexander, N. J., Clarkson, T. B.: Vasectomy increases the severity of diet-induced atherosclerosis in *Macaca fascicularis*. *Science* 1978; 201:538-541.

Alexander, N. J., Fulgham, D. L., Plunkett, E. R., Witkin, S. S.: Antisperm antibodies and circulating immune complexes of vasectomized men with and without coronary events. *American Journal of Reproductive Immunology and Microbiology* 1986; 12:38-44.

Anderson, D. J., Alexander, N. J., Fulgham, D. L., Palotay, J. L.: Spontaneous tumors in long-term-vasectomized mice: Increased incidence and association with antisperm immunity. *American Journal of Pathology* 1983; 111:129-139.

Ansbacher, R., Keung-Yueng, K., Wurster, J. C.: Sperm antibodies in vasectomized men. *Fertility and Sterility* 1972; 23:640-643.

Ansbacher, R.: Sperm antibodies after vas reanastomosis. (Letter) *The Lancet* 1977; 1:204.

102

Applebaum, P. S., Grisso, T.: Assessing patients' capacities to consent to treatment. *New England Journal of Medicine* 1988; 319:163-1638.

Bansal, N., Majumdar, Ganguly, N. K., Chakravarti, R. N.: Long term effects of vasectomy on experimental atherosclerosis in rhesus monkeys. *Australian Journal of Experimental Biology and Medical Sciences* 1986; 64:527-533.

Barclay, W. R.: Forecasting motherhood. *Journal of the American Medical Association* 1982; 247:497.

Begin v. Richmond, 555 A. 2d 363 (Wt. Sup. Ct. 1988; motions for reargument denied 1988).

Bendich, A., Borenfreund, E., Witkin, S. S. Beju, D., Huggins, P. J.: Information transfer and sperm uptake by mammalian somatic cells. In *Progress in Nucleic Acid Research and Molecular Biology*. New York: Academic Press, Inc., 17:43-45.

a. Bigazzi, P. E., Kosudo, L. L., Hsu, K. C., Andres, G. A.: Immune complex orchitis in vasectomized rabbits. *Journal of Experimental Medicine* 1976; 142:382-404.

b. Bigazzi, P. E., Kosudo, L. L., Harnick, L. L., Brown, R. C., Rose, N. R.: Antibodies to testicular antigens in vasectomized rabbits. *Clinical Immunology and Immunopathology* 1976; 5:182.

Bigazzi, P. E., Kosudo, L. L., Harnick, L. L.: Sperm autoantibodies in vasectomized rats of different inbred strains. *Science* 1977; 197:1282-1283.

Bigazzi, P. E.,: Immunologic effects of vasectomy in men and experimental animals. Chapter 41 in *Reproductive Immunology*. New York, Alan R. Liss, Inc. 1981, 474.

Bottazzo, G. F.: Cited by *The Lancet* 1992; 339:922-923.

Bowers v. Talmage, 159 So.2d 888(1963).

Bridges, F. S., Westifield, R. C.: Effects of vasectomy and exercise upon aortic extensibility, cholesterol deposition, and stainable tissue lipids. *Biology of Reproduction* 1984; 31:296-302.

Cale, A. R. J., Farouk, M., Presett, R. J., Wallace, I. W. J.: Does vasectomy accelerate testicular tumor? Importance of testicular examination before and after vasectomy. *British Medical Journal* 1990; 300:370.

Canterbury v. Spence, 150 U.S. App. D.C. 263, 464 F.2d 772 (D.C. Cir. 1972), cert. denied 409 U.S. 1064.

Casey, M. L., Byrd, W., MacDonald, P. C.: Massive amounts of immunoreactive endothelia in human seminal fluid. *Journal of Clinical Endocrinology and Metabolism* 1992; 74:223-225.

Chandra, R. K.: Immunodeficiency in undernutrition and overnutrition. *Nutrition Reviews* 1981; 39:225.

Chism, S. E., Wallis, S., Burton, R. C., Warner, N. L.: Analysis of murine oncofetal antigens as tumor-associated transplantation antigens. *Journal of Immunology* 1976; 117:1870-1877.

Coggin, J. H., Jr., Anderson, N. G.: Cancer, differentiation and embroyonic antigens: Some central problems. *Advances in Cancer Research* 1974; 9:105-165.

Corson, S. L.: Editorial comments. *Journal of Reproductive Medicine* 1993; 28:758.

Crewe, P., Dawson, L., Tidmarsh, E., Chanarin, I., Barnes, R. D.: Autoimmune implications of vasectomy in man. *Clinical and Experimental Immunology* 1976; 24:;368-369.

104

Daniel, R. K.: Microsurgery: Through the looking glass. *New England Journal of Medicine* 1979; 300:1251-1257.

Davis, J. E., de Castro, M. P. P., Mumford, S. D.: Consensus on vasectomy. *The Lancet* 1982; 2:1222.

Devlin, M. M.: Informed consent. *Journal of the American Medical Association* 1983; 249:815.

Djerassi, C.: The bitter pill. *Science* 1989; 245:356-361.

Dyer, A. R.: Cited in *Utah Science*, Winter 1991, 131.

Edey, H.: Psychological aspects of vasectomy. *Medical Counterpoint* January 1972, 19-32.

Editorial: The doctor's role in fertility regulation. *The Lancet* 1977; 1:1041.

Editorial: Safety of vasectomy. *The Lancet* 1979; 2:1057-1058.

Editorial: Vasectomy and prostate cancer. *The Lancet* 1991; 337:1445-1446.

Edwards, R. G.: Immunology of conception and pregnancy. *British Medical Bulletin* 1970; 26:72.

Fahrenbach, H. G., Alexander, N. J., Senner, J. W., et al: Effects of vasectomy on the retinal vasculature of men. *Journal of Andrology* 1980; 1:299-303.

Fisch, H., Laor, E. Barchama, N., et al.: Detection of testicular endocrine abnormalities and their correlation with serum antisperm antibodies in men following vasectomy. *Journal of Urology* 1989; 141:1129-1132.

Feature: Vasectomy and cancer. *The Lancet* 1991; 338:1586.

Fred, H. L.: Doing nothing. *Southern Medical Journal* 1992; 85:343.

Gachelin, G., Kember, R., Kelly, F., Jacob, F.: PCC4, a new cell surface antigen common to multipotential embryonal carcinoma cells, spermatozoa, and mouse early embryos. *Developmental Biology* 1977; 57:199-209.

a. Giovannucci, E., Tosteson, T. R., Speizer, F. E., et al.: A long-term study of mortality in men who have undergone vasectomy. *New England Journal of Medicine* 1992; 326:1392-1398.

b. Giovannucci, E., Speizer, F. E., Colditz, G. A.: Mortality after vasectomy. (Letter) *New England Journal of Medicine* 1992; 327:1034.

a. Giovannucci, E., Ascherio, A., Rimm, E.B., et al: A prospective cohort study of vasectomy and prostate cancer in US men. *Journal of the American Medical Association* 1993; 269: 873-877.

b. Giovannucci, E., Tosteson, T.D., Speizer, F.E., et al: A retrospective cohort study of vasectomy and prostate cancer in US men. *Journal of the American Medical Association* 1993; 269: 878-882.

Goldacre, M., Vessey, M., Clarke, J., Heasman, M.: Record linkage study of morbidity following vasectomy. In *Vasectomy: Immunologic and Pathophysiologic Effects in Animals and Man*. Academic Press, Inc., 1979; 567-579.

Goldberg, E. H., Tokuda, S.: Evidence for related antigens on sperm, tumor, and fetal cells in the mouse. *Transplantation Proceedings* 1977; 9:1363-1365.

Granai, C. O.: Ovarian cancer — unrealistic expectations. *New England Journal of Medicine* 1992; 327:197-200.

Harris, C.: Chelation: Anecdote vs science. *Medical Tribune* September 16, 1987; 14.

Harris, R. W., Scott, W. A.: Vasectomy and cancer of the cervix. *New England Journal of Medicine* 1979; 301:1064-1065.

Harris, S. J.: Feature. *The Miami Herald* September 29, 1983, A-31.

Jacob, H. S.: Complement induced granulocyte aggregation: Important in myocardial infarction and shock lung. *Journal of the American Medical Association* 1981; 245:2016.

Jarow, J. P.: Quantitative pathologic changes in the human testis after vasectomy. *New England Journal of Medicine* 1985; 313:1252-1256.

Johnson, P.: The heartless lovers of human kind. *The Wall Street Journal* January 5, 1987, 18.

Johnson, V. E.: Discussion in *Sexual Medicine Today* June 1979, 32.

Jonsen, A. R.: Do no harm. *Annals of Internal Medicine* 1978; 88:827.

Kronmal, R. A., Kriegar, J. N., Kennedy, J. W., et al: Vasectomy and urolithiasis. *The Lancet* 1988; 331:22-23.

Lapp, R. E.: Feature. *Palm Beach Post-Times* February 4, 1973.

Lauersen, N.: A closer look at sterilization. *Medical World News* May 23, 1979, 87.

Linnet, L., Hjort, T., Fogh-Anderson, P.: Association between failure to impregnate after vasovasostomy and sperm agglutinins in semen. *The Lancet* 1981; 1:117-119.

Massey, F. J., Jr., Bernstein, G. S., O'Fallon, W. M., et al: Vasectomy and health: Results from a large cohort study. *Journal of the American Medical Association* 1984; 252:1023-1029.

Matsuda, K., Masuda, A., Mathur, R., Halushka, P. V.: Testosterone increases thromboxane A2 receptor density in vascular smooth muscle cells. *Clinical Research* 1992; 40:265A.

Menge, A. C.: Antiserum inhibition of rats spermatozoal adherence ova. *Proceedings of the Society of Experimental Biology and Medicine* 1971; 138:98.

Mettlin, C., Natarajan, N., Huben, R.: Vasectomy and prostate cancer risk. *American Journal of Epidemiology* 1990; 132:1056-1061.

Mishell, D. R., Jr.: Contraception. *New England Journal of Medicine* 1989; 320:777-787.

Motulsky, A. G.: Bias ascertainment and the natural history of disease. *New England Journal of Medicine* 1978; 298:1196.

Naaby-Hansen, S.: The humoral autoimmune response to vasectomy described by immunoblotting from two-dimensional gels and demonstration of a human spermatozoa antigen immunochemically cross reactive with the D2 adhesion molecule. *Journal of Reproductive Immunology* 1990; 17:187-205.

National Research Council: *Environmental Neurotoxicology.* National Academy Press, Washington, D.C., 1991, 4.

Nienhuis, H., Goldacre, M., Seagroatt, V., Gill, L., Vessey, M.: Incidence of disease after vasectomy: a record linkage retrospective cohort study. *British Medical Journal* 1992; 304:743-746.

Nirapathpongporn, A., Huber, D. H., Krieger, J. N.: No-scalpel vasectomy at the King's birthday vasectomy festival. *The Lancet* 1990; 335:894-895.

Pabst, R., Martin, O., Lippert, H.: Is the low fertility rate after vasovasostomy caused by nerve resection during vasectomy? *Fertility and Sterility* 1979; 31:316.

Pellegrino, E. D.: Is truth telling to the patient a cultural artifact? *Journal of the American Medical Association* 1992; 268:1734-1735.

Petitti, D. B., Klein, R., Kipp, H., et al: A survey of personal habits, symptoms of illness, and histories of disease in men with and without vasectomies. *American Journal of Public Health* 1982; 72:476-480.

Phadke, A. M., Padukone, K.: Presence and significance of autoantibodies against spermatozoa in the blood of men with obstructed vas deferens. *Journal of Reproduction and Fertility* 1964; 7:163-170.

Randall, T.: United States loses lead in contraceptive choices, R & D; changes in tort liability, FDA review urged. *Journal of the American Medical Association* 1991; 268:176-179.

Ritchey, M. L., Sago, A. L., Novicki, D. E.: Effect of vasectomy on high density lipoproteins. *Journal of Urology* 1985; 133:42-44.

a. Roberts, H. J.: The syndrome of narcolepsy and diabetogenic ("functional") hyperinsulinism, with special reference to obesity, diabetes, idiopathic edema, cerebral dysrhythmias and multiple sclerosis (200 patients). *Journal of the American Geriatrics Society* 1964; 12:926-976.

b. Roberts, H. J.: Afternoon glucose tolerance testing: A key to the pathogenesis, early diagnosis and prognosis of diabetogenic hyperinsulinism. *Journal of the American Geriatrics Society* 1964; 12:423-472.

Roberts, H. J.: Obesity due to the syndrome of narcolepsy and diabetogenic hyperinsulinism: clinical and therapeutic observations on 252 patients. *Journal of the American Geriatrics Society* 1967; 15:721-743.

a. Roberts, H. J.: The value of afternoon glucose tolerance testing in the diagnosis, prognosis and rational treatment of "early chemical diabetes": a 5-year experience. *Acta Diabetologica Latina* 1968; 5:532-565.

b. Roberts, H. J.: Delayed thrombophlebitis and systemic complications after vasectomy. *Journal of the American Geriatrics Society* 1968; 16:267-280.

c. Roberts, H. J.: Voluntary sterilization in the male. (Letter). *British Medical Journal* 1968; 3:434.

Roberts, H. J.: Vasectomy. (Letter) *Perspectives in Biology and Medicine* 1970; 14 (Autumn):176.

a. Roberts, H. J.: Thrombophlebitis after vasectomy. (Letter) *New England Journal of Medicine* 1971; 284:1330.

b. Roberts, H. J.: *The Causes, Ecology and Prevention of Traffic Accidents.* Charles C Thomas, Springfield, 1971.

Roberts, H. J.: Letter. *Family Planning Perspectives* Spring 1973, 66.

a. Roberts, H. J.: *Is Vasectomy Safe? Medical, Public Health and Legal Implications* Sunshine Academic Press, West Palm Beach, 1979.

b. Roberts, H. J.: Is Vasectomy Safe? *Sexual Medicine Today* June 1979, 38.

Roberts, H. J.: Controversies and enigmas in thrombophlebitis and pulmonary embolism: Perspectives on alleged overdiagnosis. *Angiology* 1980; 31:686-699.

Roberts, H. J.: Perspectives on vitamin E as therapy. *Journal of the American Medical Association* 1981; 246:129-131.

Roberts, H. J.: The vitamin E enigma: Perspectives for physicians. Chapter 26 in *Controversies in Dermatology*, ed. by Ervin Epstein, Philadelphia, W. B. Saunders Company, 1984, 366-394.

Roberts, H. J.: Reactions attributed to aspartame-containing products: 551 cases. *Journal of Applied Nutrition* 1988; 40:85-94.

Roberts, H. J.: *Aspartame (NutraSweet®):Is It Safe?* Philadelphia, The Charles Press, 1989.

a. Roberts, H. J.: Prostate cancer and vasectomy. *Townsend Letter for Doctors* April 1992, 277-278.

b. Roberts, H. J.: Re: Toxicology of fluoride. *Townsend Letter for Doctors* July 1992, 623-624.

c. Roberts, H.J.: *Sweet'ner Dearest: Bittersweet Vignettes About Aspartame (Nutrasweet®)*. West Palm Beach, Sunshine Sentinel Press, 1992.

Rosenberg, L., Palmer, J.R., Zauber, A. G., et al: Vasectomy and the risk of prostate cancer. *American Journal of Epidemiology* 1990; 132:1051-1055.

Rümke, P.: Sperm-agglutinating autoantibodies in relation to male infertility. *Proceedings of the Royal Society of Medicine* 1968; 61:275

Rümke, P., Titus, M.: Sperm-agglutinin formation in male rats by subcutaneously injected syngeneic epididymal spermatozoa and by vasoligation or vasectomy. *Journal of Reproduction and Fertilization* 1970; 2:69.

Sackler, A. M., Wiltman, A. S., Pandhi, V., Schwartz, R.: Gonadal effects of vasectomy and vasoligation. *Science* 1973; 179:293.

Saloneu, J. T., Yla-Herttuala, S., Yamamoto, R., et al.: Autoantibody against oxidised LDL and progression of carotid atherosclerosis. *The Lancet* 1991; 339:883-887.

Salvo v. Leland Stanford, Jr., University Board of Trustees, 154 Cal. App.2d 560, 317 P.2d 170 (1957).

Samuel, T., Kolk, A. H. J., Rümke, P., Van Lis, J. M. J.: Autoimmunity to sperm antigens in vasectomized men. *Clinical and Experimental Immunology* 1975; 21:65-74.

Schloendorff v. Society of New York Hospital, 211 N.Y. 125, 105 N.E. 92(1914).

Scott v. Bradford , 606 P.2d 554 (Okla. 1979).

Selye, H.: *Discovery Processes in Modern Biology.* Chapter 12. W. R. Klemm, ed. Malabar, FL, Krieger Publishing Company, 1977.

Stein, M., Schiavi, R., C., Camerino, M.: The influence of brain and behavior on the immune system. *Science* 1976; 191:435.

Strickler, R. Z.: Tubal ligation syndrome: Does it exist? *Postgraduate Medicine* 1984; 75:233, 237.

Sullivan, M. J., Howe, G. E.: Correlation of circulating antisperm antibodies to functional success in vasovasostomy. *Journal of Urology* 1977; 117:189.

Swaw v. Klompien, 522 N.E.2d 1267 (Ill. App. Ct. 1988).

Szasz, T.: Diagnoses are not diseases. *The Lancet* 1991; 338:1574-157.

Thornhill, J. A., Butler, M., Fitzpatrick, J. M.: Could vasectomy accelerate testicular cancer? The importance of prevasectomy examination. *British Journal of Urology* 1987; 59:367.

Tung, K. S. K.: Allergic orchitis lesions are adoptively transferred from vasoligated guine pigs to syngeneic recipients. *Science,* 1978; 201:833.

Vianna, N. J.: Hodgkin's disease. *Journal of the American Medical Association* 1975; 234:1133.

Viddeleer, A. C., Nijeholt, G. A. B. L.: Lethal Fournier's gangrene following vasectomy. *Journal of Urology* 1992; 147:1613-1614.

Walker, A. M., Jick, H., Hunter, J. R., Danford, A., Rothman, K. J.: Hospitalization rates in vasectomized men. *Journal of the American Medical Association* 1981; 245:2315-2317.

Weyl, N: Aristocide as a force of history. *Intercollegiate Review* June 1967, 237.

Wilson v. Scott, 412 S.W. 2d 299(1967).

Witkin, S. S., Zelikovasky, G., Bongiovanni, A. M. et al: Sperm-related antigens, antibodies, and circulating immune complexes in sera of recently vasectomized men. *Journal of Clinical Investigation* 1982; 70:33-40.

Wolfers, D., Wolfers, H.: Vasectomania. *Family Planning Perspectives* Fall 1973, 196-199.

Wolfers, D., Wolfers, H.: *Family Planning Perspectives* 1941, Winter, 4.

INDEX

A

Advice before vasectomy 79-87
Alleged safety 20, 22, 23
  (Also see Information)
Allergic predisposition 51
  (Also see Immune Responses)
Allergies after vasectomy 21, 51, 60-62
Alternatives 74-77, 80-84
Angina pectoris 65-67
Anguish of parents 9
Antibodies 13-14, 44-51, 57-58, 67-69,
  83 (Also see Immune Response.s)
Antigens 44-51
Arthritis 16, 17, 57, 58
Arthropathy (See Arthritis)
Aspartame 30
Arrhythmias (cardiac) 68
Association for Voluntary Sterilization 35
Asthma 60
Atherosclerosis 65-67

B

"Brainwashing" 30
(Also see Disinformation)

C

Cancer after vasectomy
  Computer searches 22
  General 27, 69-72
  Prostate 14, 22, 69-72
  Testicle 28, 71
Cholesterol 66, 67
Confusion 68
Contraceptive counseling 74, 80-87
Contraceptive drugs ("the pill") 81

D

Dermatitis 60, 68
  (Also see Allergies)
Disinformation 14, 22, 23, 29
  (Also see Information, Informed
  Consent)
  Patient education 14, 29
  Physician denial 30, 31

Drowsiness 58
  (Also see narcolepsy)

E

Emotional disturbances 62, 63
Epidemiology 34-36, 75
Epilepsy 68
Ethical considerations 14, 15, 80-87
  (Also see Informed Consent)

Failure to inquire 25, 26
Failure to obtain proper consent 74-77
Failure to reveal past history 26
Family planning 80-87
Federal encouragement 40
Fever 68
Flawed research protocols 16, 26-28
Followup deficiencies
  Cancer 69-72
  Resistance 15
  Routine inquiry by surgeons 23

G

Genocide 86

H

Hair loss 68
Headache 59
HIV infection 57
Hives 60-62
Hormonal changes 63-65
Hypertension 68
Hyperthyroidism (Graves' disease) 17, 68
Hypoglycemia 51, 59, 60

I

Ignorance of literature by professionals
  14, 24
Immune responses to vasectomy 13-16,
  44-51 (Also see Antibodies)
Immune cascade 44, 45
Immune complexes 47-49, 58, 66, 67
Immunologic exhaustion 25
Infection 56, 57
Information blackout 19-31
  Failure to publish 11-9
  Obstacles 22-31
  Pleas for 16,17
  Shortcomings of pamphlets 76
  Shortcomings of professionals 14,
  15, 23-25, 74-77
Informed consent 14, 15, 74-77, 82-84
  (Also see Ethics)
  Consequences of absence 38, 39
  Doctrine 75-77
Insurance as a factor 40
In vitro fertilization 84
Intrauterine devices (IUD's) 80, 81

K

Kidney
  Infection 56, 57
  Inflammation 68
  Stones 65

Leg cramps 68
Leukemia 69, 71
Litigation 26, 74-77
    (Also see Medicolegal)
Lung
    Cancer 71, 72
    Inflammation 68
Lymph node enlargement 68

M

Magnitude of vasectomy 13, 14, 33-36
    (Also see Vasectomy Crusade)
Medical complications 53-72
Medicolegal 26, 40, 74-77
    (Also see Litigation)
Migraine 59
Multiple sclerosis 30, 58, 59
Myocardial infarction 65-67

N

Narcolepsy 58

O

Obstacles 22-31
    (Also see Resistance)

P

Pain—testicles, scrotum 68, 75-76
Pancreatitis 68
Peptic ulcer 68
Perspectives 15, 16, 79-87
Physical activity 51
Polyneuropathy 68
Population Reports 25, 39
Prostate cancer after vasectomy 14, 22, 69-72
Prostatitis 56, 57
Publication deficiencies 24-30
    (Also see Information and Resistance)
Pulmonary embolism 54-56
    (Also see Thrombophlebitis)

Q

Questionnaire followup - Appendix A
Questions-and-Answers pamphlets 29, 76

R

Rashes 60-62, 68
Resistance to followup 14-16, 22-31
Resistance to publication 26
Restless legs 68
Reversal of vasectomy 15-17, 83
    (See Vasovasostomy)
Resistance to obtain data 29, 30

S

Sarcoidosis 68
Sexual inadequacy 63-65
Single males 82
Social repercussions 36, 79-87
Sperm banking 84
Sterility
    Before vasectomy (unrecognized) 80
    After reversal 15, 83
Superspecialization influence 24

T

Thrombophlebitis 31, 54-56
    (Also see Pulmonary Embolism)
Tonsillectomy 51
Trivialization of findings 28
Tubal ligation 84
Tumors 69-72
    (Also see Cancer)

U

Urologist "truth squads" 23

V

Vasectomania 35, 36, 38, 39
Vasectomy
    Failure 77
    Immune responses 43-51
    Liberalized requirements 40
    Medical complications 53-72
    Operative techniques 12, 13
Vasectomy complications 53-72
    Contributory factors 51
Vasectomy crusade 37-41
Vasovasostomy (reversal) 15-17, 68, 69, 83
    Failure to relieve pain 15, 17, 68, 69
    High cost 15
    Persistent postoperative infertility 64, 65, 83

W

Weight loss 68

Z

Zero Population Growth (ZPG) 13, 23, 38, 85